OKANAGAN UNIV/COLLEGE LIBRARY

02800639

P9-DTC-617

K

PT 82.8 .A49 196

BRITISH COLUMBIA

ADVANCED PRACTICE NURSING

A Guide to Professional Development

2nd Edition

Mariah Snyder, PhD, RN, FAAN
Michaelene P. Mirr, PhD, RN, CS
Editors

 Springer Series: Advanced Practice Nursing

Copyright © 1999 by Springer Publishing Company, Inc.

All rights reserved.

No part of this publication may be reproduced, stored in a retrieval system, or transmitted in any form or by any means, electronic, mechanical, photocopying, recording, or otherwise, without the prior permission of Springer Publishing Company, Inc.

Springer Publishing Company, Inc.
536 Broadway
New York, NY   10012-3955

Cover design by James Scotto-Lovino
Acquisitions Editor: Ruth Chasek
Production Editor: Sandi Borger

99 00 01 02 03 / 5 4 3 2 1

Library of Congress Cataloging-in-Publication Data

Advanced practice nursing : a guide to professional development /
   Mariah Snyder, and Michaelene Mirr, editors. — 2nd ed.
     p. cm. — (Springer series on advanced practice nursing)
     Includes bibliographical references and index.
     ISBN 0-8261-1281-1 (hardcover)
     1. Nurse practitioners. 2. Primary care (Medicine) I. Snyder,
  Mariah. II. Mirr, Michaelene P. III. Series.
     [DNLM: 1. Nurse Clinicians. 2. Nurse Practitioners. 3. Nurse
  Anesthetists. 4. Nurse Midwives. WY 128 A244 1999]
  RT82.8.A49   1999
  610.73'06'92—dc21
  DNLM/DLC
  for Library of Congress   99-27973
                                      CIP

Printed in the United States of America

Springer Series on Advanced Practice Nursing

Terry T. Fulmer, PhD, RN, FAAN, Series Editor

New York University School of Nursing

Advisory Board:
Joyce Anastasi, RN, PhD;
Susan Kelley, RN, PhD, FAAN;
Tish Knobf, MSN, RN, FAAN;
Mairead Hickey, RN, PhD

Mariah Snyder, PhD, RN, FAAN, received her bachelor's degree in nursing from the College of St. Teresa, Winona, MN, her master's degree in nursing (as a medical-surgical clinical nurse specialist) from the University of Pennsylvania, Philadelphia, and her doctorate in education from the University of Minnesota, Minneapolis. Dr. Snyder is currently a professor of nursing at the University of Minnesota and coordinates the gerontological nursing area of study that prepares advanced practice nurses. She has addressed national and international audiences and has published extensively on topics about nursing care of persons with chronic health problems, the efficacy of nursing interventions, stress and coping, and nursing diagnoses.

Michaelene Pheifer Mirr, RN, PhD, CS, received her master's degree in nursing from the University of Wisconsin-Madison and her doctoral degree in nursing from the University of Minnesota. She is currently a Professor in Adult Health Nursing at the University of Wisconsin-Eau Claire. She is certified as a gerontological nurse practitioner and has a part-time affiliation with a local primary care clinic. She also works as an on-call staff nurse in an acute care facility. Her recent publications are in the areas of clinical neuroscience nursing and advanced nursing practice.

CONTENTS

LIST OF CONTRIBUTORS

Melissa Avery PhD, RN, CNM
Assistant Professor
School of Nursing
University of Minnesota
Minneapolis, MN

**Sheila Corcoran-Perry PhD,
RN, FAAN**
Professor
School of Nursing
University of Minnesota
Minneapolis, MN

**Kathleen Fagerlund PhD, RN,
CRNA**
Program Director, School of
Anesthesia
Minneapolis Veterans Affairs
Medical Center
Minneapolis, MN

Helen Hansen, PhD, RN
Assistant Professor
School of Nursing
University of Minnesota
Minneapolis, MN

Rita Kisting Sparks PhD, RN
Professor
Department of Nursing
University of Wisconsin-Eau
Claire
Eau Claire, WI

Kathleen Krichbaum PhD, RN
Associate Professor
School of Nursing
University of Minnesota
Minneapolis, MN

Marsha L. Lewis PhD, RN
Assistant Professor
School of Nursing
University of Minnesota
Minneapolis, MN

Linda Lindeke PhD, RN, CPNP
Assistant Professor
School of Nursing
University of Minnesota
Minneapolis, MN

Ruth Lindquist PhD, RN
Associate Professor
School of Nursing
University of Minnesota
Minneapolis, MN

Michaelene Mirr PhD, RN, CS
Professor
Department of Nursing
University of Wisconsin-Eau
   Claire
Eau Claire, WI

Deborah Monicken MS, CRRN, CS
Clinical Nurse Specialist
Minneapolis Veterans Affairs
   Medical Center
Minneapolis, MN

Suzanne Narayan PhD, RN
Professor
Metropolitan State University
St. Paul, MN

Margot Nelson PhD, RN
Associate Professor
Department of Nursing
Augustana College
Sioux Falls, SD 57197

Jennifer Peters PhD, RN
Assistant Educational Specialist
School of Nursing
University of Minnesota
Minneapolis, MN

**Mariah Snyder PhD, RN,
   FAAN**
Professor and Division Head for
   Adult, Gerontological, and
   Psychiatric/Mental Health
   Nursing
School of Nursing
University of Minnesota
Minneapolis, MN

Yueh-hsia Tseng MS, RN
Doctoral Student
University of Minnesota
Minneapolis, MN

Shigeaki Watanuki MS, RN
Doctoral Student
University of Minnesota
Minneapolis, MN
1064 27th Ave. SE, #A
Minneapolis, MN 55414

**Pamela J. Weiss PhD, RN, Dipl.
   Ac., L.Ac.**
Educations Specialist, School of
   Nursing
Center for Spirituality and
   Healing
University of Minnesota
Minneapolis, MN

**M. Cecilia Wendler RN, MS,
   CCRN, Doctoral Student**
Assistant Professor
University of Wisconsin-Eau
   Claire
Eau Claire, WI

**Mary Zwygart-Stauffacher
   PhD, RN, CS, GNP/GCNS**
Associate Professor
School of Nursing
University of Minnesota
Minneapolis, MN

PREFACE

If one thing has characterized the delivery of health care during the past several decades, it has been change. Technological advances are now being tempered with the increasing consumer demand for complementary/alternative therapies and caring. Efforts to control the escalating health care costs has resulted in attention being given to which health professional can most effectively and efficiently deliver specific care in a specific setting. This attention has resulted in greater use of nurses, particularly advanced practice nurses (APNs).

The more visible roles APNs are assuming in the delivery of care has been the focus of numerous media features. Although progress has been made in removing barriers that prevented APNs from utilizing all of their knowledge and skills, ongoing efforts are needed so that APNs can make even greater contributions to improving the health status of clients in a variety of settings. It is imperative not only that students in advanced practice nursing education programs be provided with content and experiences that relate to the medical aspect of care, but that this content and these experiences emphasize the need for evidence-based practice that is provided within a nursing perspective.

During the past decade there has been a growing trend toward educators and practitioners in the four advanced practice roles (certified registered nurse anesthetist [CRNA], certified nurse-midwife [CNM], nurse practitioner [NP], and clinical nurse specialist [CNS]) working together to influence health policy and legislation. Also, a common core of knowledge for the four roles has been identified. Content in this book is applicable for students in educational programs for any of the four APN roles. The content presented is not setting- or role-specific, but rather addresses the competencies identified by the National Organization of Nurse Practitioner Faculty (NONPF) and the American Association of Colleges of Nursing (AACN). A brief overview of each of the four roles and the historical context within which they developed provides students with an understanding of the richness of advanced practice nursing.

Contributors bring perspectives from a wide variety of practice backgrounds and scholarly endeavors. Their current, active involvement in the delivery of care ensures that the content presented is critical for students as they embark on a new career as APNs.

Content in all of the chapters has been updated to reflect current research, health policy, and advances in nursing. Several new chapters (including complementary therapies and ethical issues) have been added to reflect issues in the current health care system. Greater attention has been given to inclusion of content that is relevant for CRNAs and CNMs. Content is presented on the APN as consultant, communicator, advocate, care manager, change agent, and educator. Additionally, attention is given to the expanding opportunities available for APNs.

We are confident that the 21st century will see nurses, and particularly APNs, assuming more responsibility for the delivery of quality, cost-effective care to patients in multiple settings and from diverse cultural/ethnic groups. It is our hope that this text will assist students in APN programs to acquire knowledge about the advanced practice nursing role and to be better positioned to make significant contributions that will have an impact on patient outcomes and that will advance the profession of nursing.

Mariah Snyder
Michaelene Mirr

Chapter 1

ADVANCED PRACTICE NURSING: AN OVERVIEW

Mariah Snyder PhD, RN, FAAN
Michaelene P. Mirr, PhD, RN
Linda Lindeke, PhD, RN
Kathleen Fagerlund, PhD, RN
Melissa Avery, PhD, RN
Yueh-hsia Tseng, MS, RN

Practice of nurses with formal education beyond the basic preparation has a long history in nursing. However, the preparation, certification, and licensing of these practitioners has varied greatly across areas of specialization. A number of recent occurrences have prompted nursing to identify commonalities that exist in nurses who have post-basic preparation. The term "advanced practice nurses" has been chosen to denote nurses who have formal post-baccalaureate preparation (American Association of Colleges of Nursing [AACN], 1997; American Nurses Association [ANA], 1996). Advanced practice nurses encompass four groups: nurse-midwives, nurse anesthetists, nurse practitioners, and clinical nurse specialists. Originally the term was used to designate a possible merger of the nurse practitioner and clinical nurse specialist groups. However, it is now used in a broader context.

1

As noted, a number of factors have focused nursing's attention on delineating what constitutes advanced practice nursing. Direct reimbursement for nursing services by third-party payers is increasing. This requires that nursing be able to specify the preparation of these practitioners and that a common name is used to designate these practitioners. State boards of nursing are giving attention to guaranteeing patients that nurses who state they have advanced preparation have certain expertise and skills; this group has devoted time to exploring second-level licensure, and in so doing has explored the commonalities of nurses with advanced education for practice. Additionally, nursing organizations such as AACN, ANA, National Organization of Nurse Practitioner Faculties (NONPF) and numerous speciality organizations have sought to define advanced practice nursing and the educational preparation needed to practice in this role.

Although recent intense attention has been given to advanced practice nursing, the endeavors of a number of early nursing leaders planted the seed for the evolution of advanced practice nursing. Florence Nightingale emphasized the need for nurses to collect and analyze data about the efficacy of care provided to patients. Evaluation of care is a key characteristic of advanced practice nurses (APNs). Awareness and participation in health policy and legislation is another characteristic of APNs; Lavinia Dock laid the foundation for nurses' participation in the political and legislative process. Autonomy is a third characteristic of APNs. Early nurse leaders such as Lillian Wald of the Henry Street Settlement House and Mary Breckenridge, who founded the Frontier Nursing Service that provided midwifery services, sought to increase nurses' autonomy in the delivery of patient care.

Description of the four groups that comprise advanced practice nursing and their evolution, commonalities possessed by all APNs, and issues related to titling, licensing, and certification will be discussed in this chapter.

ADVANCED PRACTICE NURSING

Numerous definitions of advanced practice nursing exist. In *Nursing's Social Policy Statement* the ANA (1995) defined advanced practice registered nurses as "having acquired the knowledge base and practice experience to prepare them for specialization, expansion, and advancement in practice" (p. 9). Specialization is concentrating or delimiting one's focus to part of the whole field of nursing. Expansion refers to the acquisition of new practice knowledge and skills, including knowledge and skills legitimizing role autonomy within areas of practice that overlap traditional boundaries of medical practice. Advancement involves both specialization and expansion and is characterized by the integration of theoretical, research-based, and practical knowledge that occurs as a part of graduate education in nursing (p. 14). This definition refers to nurses engaged in clinical practice and not nurses with advanced preparation for administration, education, or research (ANA, 1995).

Only recently has the expectation been that the majority of APNs receive their education within a master's or doctoral nursing program. Except for clinical nurse specialists, the educational preparation for many nurse-midwives, nurse anesthetists, and nurse practitioners was outside of graduate nursing programs. Now, Nurse Practitioners (NPs) must receive their education in graduate master's programs in nursing. Many nurse anesthetists receive preparation in graduate nursing programs, but the certification only requires a master's degree which does not necessarily have to be in nursing. The majority of certified nurse-midwives (CNM) are prepared in graduate nursing programs. Moving education of APNs within master's programs of nursing has facilitated the adoption of a common expectations for CNMs, Certified Registered Nurse Anesthetists (CRNAs), NPs, and Clinical Nurse Specialist (CNSs).

Each of the four groups included within the definition of APNs has evolved along different paths and during different time frames. Because of the historical underpinnings, each of the APN groups has developed a strong sense of history, with members having a strong allegiance to their title and their group. This allegiance has been a barrier to the development of one APN role as members cling to their particular form of education, history, and title. However, significant progress has and continues to be made in identifying commonalities.

Nurse-Midwives

Certified Nurse-Midwives (CNMs) are defined by the American College of Nurse-Midwives (ACNM) as individuals educated in the two disciplines of nursing and midwifery and who possess evidence of certification according to the requirements of ACNM (ACNM, 1997a). Nurse-midwifery practice

> is the independent management of women's health care, focusing particularly on pregnancy, childbirth, the postpartum period, care of the newborn, and the family planning and gynecological needs of women. The CNM practices within a health care system that provides for consultation, collaborative management or referral as indicated by the health status of the client. CNMs practice in accord with the Standards for the Practice of Nurse-Midwifery, as defined by the ACNM" (ACNM, 1997c, p. 1).

In addition to providing prenatal care and managing labor and births, nurse-midwives also provide care for well women. This care includes family planning services, other gynecological needs, and peri-and post-menopausal care throughout the life cycle.

Nurse-midwives believe strongly in supporting natural processes and not intervening unless there is a clear indication. This belief and others are reflected in the ACNM philosophy statement.

> Nurse-midwives believe that every individual has the right to safe, satisfying health care with respect for human dignity and cultural variations. We further support each person's right to self-determination, to complete information and to active participation in all aspects of care. We believe the normal processes of pregnancy and birth can be enhanced through education, health care and supportive intervention. Nurse-midwifery care is focused on the needs of the individual and family for physical care, emotional and social support and active involvement of significant others according to cultural values and personal preferences. The practice of nurse-midwifery encourages continuity of care; emphasizes safe, competent clinical care; advocates non-intervention in normal processes; and promotes health education for women throughout the childbearing cycle." (ACNM, 1989, p. 1).

Midwifery is a very old profession and, in fact, is mentioned in the Bible. The practice of midwifery as it was known declined in the 18th and 19th centuries, and obstetrics developed as a medical specialty. In 1925, Mary Breckenridge established the Frontier Nursing Service (FNS) in Kentucky and was the first nurse to practice as a nurse-midwife in the United States. She received her midwifery education in England and returned with other British nurse-midwives to set up a system of care similar to that which she had observed in Scotland. FNS was begun to respond to individuals who were without adequate health care. The nurse-midwives at FNS provided maternal and infant care and effectively demonstrated quality care and significantly improved outcomes. The first U.S. nurse-midwifery education program was started at the Maternity Center Association, Lobenstein Clinic, in New York City in 1932. The American College of Nurse-Midwives was incorporated in 1955. Nurse-midwifery practice grew slowly until the late 1960s and early 1970s when nurse-midwifery experienced increased acceptance as a profession and an increase in consumer demand for nurse-midwives and the kind of care they provided (Varney, 1997).

In the 1970s, national accreditation of nurse-midwifery educational programs and national certification of nurse-midwives was begun by ACNM. The accreditation process is recognized by the United States Department of Education and certification, now conducted by the ACNM Certification Corporation, is recognized by the National Commission of Health Certifying Agencies (Varney, 1997). There are over 6000 CNMs in the U S, and in 1996 they managed over 216,000 births, or 5.6% of U.S. births (Ventura, Martin, Curtin, & Matthewa, 1998). Nurse-midwives have direct third-party reimbursement and prescriptive authority in a majority of states.

The ACNM document Core Competencies for Basic Midwifery Practice describes the skills and knowledge that are fundamental to the practice of a new graduate of an ACNM accredited education program. These competencies guide curricular development in nurse-midwifery programs and are utilized in the accreditation process. Categories of competencies are professional responsibilities; the midwifery management process; the childbearing family, including pre-conception care, care of the child-bearing woman, newborn care; and primary care of women including health promotion and disease prevention, management of common health problems, family planning/gynecologic care, perimenopause and post-menopause (ACNM, 1997a).

Nurse-midwifery education began with certificate programs and has progressed to primarily, but not entirely, graduate education. There are presently 47 nurse-midwifery programs in the United States. All but seven are in master's programs of nursing; a majority of the certificate programs have an affiliation with a graduate program.

Nurse-midwives in the US have consistently demonstrated their care results in excellent outcomes and client satisfaction. These outcomes include those of the large proportion of undeserved, uninsured, low-income, minority and otherwise vulnerable women for whom CNMs provide care. Recently, researchers have demonstrated lower cesarean section rates and outcomes comparable to a private obstetrics practice in a nurse-midwifery practice caring for undeserved women (Blanchette, 1995), and fewer interventions, including a lower cesarean section rate, for nurse-midwifery clients compared with similar low risk women cared for by family physicians and obstetricians (Rosenblatt et al, 1997). A study at the National Center for Health Statistics demonstrated significantly lower risks of neonatal mortality, low birth weight, infant mortality and a signficantly higher mean birth weight in births attended by nurse-midwives compared with those attended by physicians. These comparisons controlled for medical and sociodemographic risks (MacDorman & Singh, 1998).

Over the 70+-year history of nurse-midwifery in the United States, a strong base of support, documented by research, has been developed. The number of educational programs and practitioners have grown substantially. As health care dollars are more carefully allocated and specific outcomes are measured more closely, certified nurse-midwives should continue to play a primary role in providing quality care.

Nurse Anesthetists

Modern nurse anesthesia traces its roots to the last two decades of the 1800s, where records indicate that nurses were often asked to administer anesthesia. The practice was so common, in fact, that in her 1893 textbook entitled *Nursing: Its Principles and Practices for Hospital and Private Use,* Isabel Adams Hampton Robb included a chapter on the administration of anesthesia. By 1912, a formal course in anesthesia had been developed in Springfield, Illinois, by Mother Magdalene Weidlocher. Nurse anesthetists at St. Mary's Hospital in Rochester, Minnesota, became well known for their expertise in administration of anesthesia (Bankert, 1989). Alice McGaw, one of the early nurse anesthetists for the Drs. Mayo, published several papers in the early 1900s reporting on the thousands of anesthetics administered with ether and/or chloroform—all "without a death attributable to the anesthesia" (Bankert, 1989, p. 31).

A Certified Registered Nurse Anesthetist (CRNA) is a registered nurse who is educationally prepared to provide anesthesia and anesthesia-related services in collaboration with other health care professionals. The practice of nurse anesthesia is a specialty within the profession of nursing, and in all 50 states CRNAs are recognized by state licensing or regulatory agencies, primarily boards of nursing (Jordan, 1994).

According to the American Association of Nurse Anesthetists (AANA), the CRNA scope of practice includes, but is not limited to:

1. Performing and documenting a pre-anesthetic assessment and evaluation of the patient, including requesting consultations and diagnostic studies: selecting, obtaining, ordering, and administering pre-anesthetic medications and fluids; and obtaining informed consent for anesthesia.

2. Developing and implementing an anesthetic plan.

3. Initiating the anesthetic technique which may include: general, regional, local and sedation.

4. Selecting, applying, and inserting appropriate non-invasive and invasive monitoring modalities for continuous evaluation of the patient's physical status.

5. Selecting, obtaining, and administering the anesthetics, adjuvant and accessory drugs, and fluids necessary to manage the anesthetic.

6. Managing a patient's airway and pulmonary status using current practice modalities.

7. Facilitating emergence and recovery from anesthesia by selecting, obtaining, ordering and administering medications, fluids, and ventilatory support.

8. Discharging the patient from a postanesthesia care area and providing postanesthesia follow-up evaluation and care.

9. Implementing acute and chronic pain management modalities.

10. Responding to emergency situations by providing airway management, administration of emergency fluids and drugs, and using basic or advanced cardiac life support techniques. (AANA, 1996, p. 1)

Nurse anesthesia educational programs are a minimum of 24 months in length and exist in a master's degree framework. In 1998, approximately 40% of nurse anesthesia educational programs were housed within or affiliated with graduate nursing programs. The other programs offer a variety of master's degrees, including majors such as nurse anesthesiology, biology, health science, or anesthesiology education. All programs are accredited by the Council on Accreditation for Nurse Anesthesia Educational Programs (COA), which in turn is recognized by the U.S. Department of Education and the Commission on Recognition of Postsecondary Accreditation (CORPA). This formal accreditation program was begun in 1952. While most programs exceed these requirements, all nurse anesthesia programs, regardless of the master's degree offered, provide a minimum of: 45 hours of professional aspects, 135 hours of anatomy, physiology, and pathophysiology, 45 hours of chemistry and physics, 90 hours of anesthesia principles, and 45 hours of clinical and literature review conferences. In addition to these classroom hours, the administration of at least 450 anesthetics is required (AANA, 1992).

To become a CRNA, a student must successfully complete the Certification Examination administered by the Council on Certification of

Nurse Anesthetists (CCNA). Because CRNAs must graduate from a COA-accredited educational program and pass the Certification Exam to practice, the public can be assured that a CRNA has a certain standard level of expertise. In spite of this standardization, clinical practice opportunities vary considerably for CRNAs. Approximately 80% of the CRNAs practice in anesthesia care teams with anesthesiologists, and the other 20% practice independently as sole anesthesia providers in hospitals or outpatient clinics, providing the entire range of anesthesia options for their clients. CRNAs practicing in anesthesia care teams may find their clinical privileges limited to certain anesthesia modalities (e.g., general and intravenous anesthesia, but not regional anesthesia).

The Omnibus Budget Reconciliation Act of 1986 (cited in Jordan, 1994) granted CRNAs the right to be reimbursed directly by Medicare, giving CRNAs new practice options. Because CRNAs function as sole anesthesia providers in over 70% of rural hospitals (AANA, 1998), the AANA has made it a priority to assure that health care plans cannot exclude providers based solely on their license or credentials.

CRNAs are legally liable for their own actions and are supportive of legislation that eliminates the requirement for physician supervision of CRNA practice. A current proposal by the Health Care Financing Administration (HCFA) eliminates the federal physician supervision requirement and defers to state law. While the HCFA proposal is controversial, it affirms the quality of anesthesia care provided by CRNAs in the United States.

Nurse Practitioners

Nurse practitioners (NPs) have been defined by the ANA (1996) in the following manner:

> The nurse practitioner provides comprehensive health assessments, determines diagnosis, plans and prescribes treatments and manages health care regimens in a variety of settings for individuals, families, and communities. This role includes promotion of wellness, prevention of illness and injury and management of acute and chronic conditions (p. 4).

Nurse practitioners have traditionally been defined as primary care providers. However, NPs are now functioning in tertiary care settings.

The shortage of physicians during the 1960s led to the development of the nurse practitioner role. The nurse practitioner movement began at the University of Colorado; Loretta Ford and Henry Silver began a post-baccalaureate program to prepare nurses for an expanded role in care of children. Ford and Silver (1967) noted that the key to their program was the "development of the nurse's ability to judge levels of wellness so that appropriate nursing action may be taken toward health-oriented goals" (p. 45). The purpose of the first nurse practitioner demonstration project was to implement a new role for nurses to evaluate this role for its effectiveness in improving the safety, efficacy, and quality of health care for children and families (Ford, 1979). Although the project's initial focus was on children and families, Ford noted that she was confident that nurses could be educated to meet the health needs of community-dwelling persons across the life span. Nurses in the Colorado program received 4 months of intensive didactic education in which assessment skills and growth and development were emphasized. The nurses then completed a 20-month precepted clinical in a community-based setting.

Following Colorado's lead, many schools initiated educational programs to prepare nurse practitioners. Many of these were certificate programs admitting nurses with varying levels of educational preparation. The growth of the nurse practitioner movement was facilitated by findings from an interdisciplinary committee of health providers convened by the Secretary of the Department of Health, Education, and Welfare in 1971. This committee concluded that in order to provide adequate health care to all United States citizens, the role of nursing had to be expanded (Kalisch & Kalisch, 1986). These recommendations served as the impetus for increased federal funding for nurse practitioner programs. Although the initial goal was to have nurse practitioners prepared within master's programs, societal demand for nurse practitioners led to a proliferation of postbaccalaureate continuing education programs rather than graduate education (Ford, 1979; Kitzman, 1983). Federal funding for nurse practitioner programs also prompted the initiation of numerous postbaccalaureate and graduate nurse practitioner programs. The length of NP programs varied from a few weeks to 2 years, with many certificate programs being 9 to 12 months in length.

The proliferation of postbaccalaureate rather than graduate programs for the education of NPs was partially due to the resistance of graduate nursing programs to recognize NPs as being a legitimate part of nursing. A number of nursing leaders termed NPs as "physician-extenders" and did not view NP practice as being "nursing." This lack of enthusiasm for NP education exhibited by numerous graduate education programs may also have been fostered by the fact the NP movement grew out of a collaborative nurse-physician effort rather than being solely initiated by nurses. The NP curricula tended to be based on the medical model rather than a nursing framework.

There are over 53,753 NPs who have been prepared in a multitude of specialties including pediatrics, adult health, acute care, neonatal, gerontology, women's health, and family. After completing their education, NPs take a certification examination. (Certification is needed for NPs to receive third-party reimbursement.) Certification examinations are offered by a variety of bodies: the American Nurses Credentialing Center, the American Academy of Nurse Practitioners, the National Certification Board of Pediatric Nurse Practitioners and Nurses, and the National Certification Corporation for the obstetric, gynecologic, and nursing specialties. In most instances, certification needs to be renewed every 5 years. This requires documentation of continuing education and practice.

Changes in reimbursement policy that allows for direct reimbursement of NPs, the rapid increase in managed care as a mechanism to control health care costs, and the growing recognition of the significant contributions of NPs to positive patient outcomes has resulted in a rapid increase in the number of NP programs. Currently, 295 schools of nursing prepare nurse practitioners (AACN, 1998). This rapid increase in NP programs has raised concerns about the production of too many NPs. Another concern is the availability of qualified faculty to teach in NP programs. The Pew Health Professions Commission (1994a) noted an increased demand for master's-prepared nurses. New roles for NPs continue to evolve. Thus, concerns about overproduction do not appear, at least within the near future, to be well-founded.

Great variation in the length of educational programs for NPs, the content presented, and the amount of clinical experience has existed since 1967. These discrepancies prompted the NONPF to develop curriculum guidelines and program standards for NP education (NONPF, 1995). These guidelines make a major contribution to standardizing NP preparation and ultimately NP practice.

NPs have a relatively short history in the health care delivery system. However, in this short period of time they have gained the respect of many health professionals and of their patients. Recently, television and lay publications have featured NPs and the significant contributions that they are making to improve health. In many instances care has been for persons in rural areas, inner city, and other vulnerable groups. NPs have established themselves as an integral part of the health care system.

Clinical Nurse Specialists

The ANA (1996) defined clinical nurse specialists (CNSs) in the following manner:

> The clinical nurse specialist is a clinical expert who provides direct patient care services including health assessment, diagnosis, health promotive and preventive interventions and management of health problems in a specialized area of nursing practice. The clinical nurse specialist promotes the improvement of nursing care through education, consultation, research, and in the role of change agent in the health care system (p. 3).

CNSs have traditionally worked in hospitals, but they now practice in many settings such as nursing homes, schools, home care, and hospice.

Like NPs, CNSs developed after World War II. Initially, specialization for nurses was in the functional areas of administration and education. Recognizing the need to have highly qualified nurses directly involved in patient care, the concept of clinical nurse specialists emerged. Reiter has been credited with first using the term "nurse clinician" in 1943 to designate a specialist in nursing practice (Reiter, 1966). The first master's program in a clinical specialty in nursing was developed by Hildegarde Peplau at Rutgers University in 1954. This program prepared psychiatric clinical nurse specialists.

As with the NP movement, the availability of federal funds for graduate nursing education programs and the Professional Traineeship Program that provided stipends for students resulted in the development of numerous graduate programs offering CNS areas of study. Currently, 306 schools offer master's programs (National League for Nursing, 1997). Except for the curriculum proposed for graduate clinical education by the American Association of Colleges of Nursing, which will be addressed in the next section, no uniform curriculum has been proposed for CNS education.

The development and use of complex technology in the management of patients in hospitals and intricate surgical procedures has resulted in an increase in the acuity of hospital patients. Thus, there is a need for nurses with advanced knowledge and expertise to be integrally involved in working with staff to assess, plan, implement, and evaluate care for these patients. Many hospitals have placed CNSs in the role of case manager to coordinate the care of patients with high acuity during their hospital experience (Wells, Erickson, & Spinella, 1996). CNSs have also been used as discharge planners to work with staff to plan post-hospital care for patients who have complex health problems (Naylor et al., 1994; Neidlinger, Scroggins, & Kennedy, 1987). Naylor and colleagues reported that use of gerontological CNSs as discharge planners resulted in fewer readmissions of elderly cardiac patients.

Since its inception, the CNS role has suffered from role ambiguity (Rasch & Frauman, 1996; Redekopp, 1997). While the initial vision for CNSs was for them to be integrally involved in patient care for a specific patient population, CNSs have assumed many other roles, such as staff and patient educator, consultant, supervisor, project director, and more recently, case manager. Redekopp notes that is difficult for a CNS to precisely describe the role to others, as the role is continually changing to meet the health needs of a changing population within an ever-changing health care system. Role ambiguity has made it difficult to measure the impact that CNSs have on patient outcomes. Thus, when budgetary crises occur within hospitals, CNSs have frequently had to fight to maintain their positions as outcome data to support the positive impact of their practice does not exist.

Numerous CNS specialities and subspecialties exist. These include psychiatric/mental health nursing, adult health, gerontology, oncology, pediatrics, cardiovascular, neuroscience, rehabilitation, pulmonary, renal, diabetes, and palliative care. These are only a few of the many, many specialties that have emerged. Numerous organizations offer certification examinations for CNSs. However, some organizations do not require a master's degree to become certified as a clinical nurse specialist. The ANCC began offering certification examinations in 1974. Because many CNSs have not sought third-party reimbursement, many CNSs have not taken the certification examination for their specialty. With changes in state nursing practice acts and the increase in third-party payment for advanced practice nurses, the number of certified CNS will most likely increase.

In the late 1980s and early 1990s, many discussions and debates occurred about the merging of the CNS and NP roles (Page & Arena, 1994). Several studies were conducted comparing the knowledge and skills of these two advanced practice roles (Elder & Bullough, 1990; Fenton & Brykczynski, 1993; Forbes, Rafson, Spross, & Kozlowski, 1990). Findings indicated many similarities in the educational preparation of these two groups of APNs. Many CNSs viewed the proposed merger as the demise of the CNS role. NPs were concerned that they would need to abandon the title of NP, a title that had become familiar to many patients and health professionals. A new organization, the National Association of Clinical Nurse Specialists, was formed to assist CNSs and to provide a vehicle to publicize the many contributions that CNSs have and continue to make providing quality patient care. Vollman and Stewart (1996) noted that we cannot afford not to have CNSs.

CHARACTERISTICS OF APNs

The debate about the merger of the CNS and NP roles was one impetus for nursing organizations to give attention to what constitutes the educational preparation of APNs and what common characteristics transcend all four groups. Cronenwett (1995) noted:

> During this time when the walls that divide inpatient, outpatient, primary, tertiary, and community care are coming down, society should expect that the nursing profession will prepare and regulate advanced nursing practice for the good of patient care and society as a whole. To do so, schools with clinical practice graduate programs must create a consistent product; professional credentialing bodies must use consistent criteria to acknowledge advanced practice knowledge and expertise; and state boards of nursing must give legal recognition for advanced practice to these same nurses. (p. 117)

Numerous other nursing leaders have acknowledged the need for unity within advanced practice nursing so that nursing can more easily work with legislators, political bodies, third-party payers, and society (Long, 1994; Rasch & Frauman, 1996).

Traditionally, four roles have been identified for the advanced practice nurse: patient care, educator, consultant, and researcher (Hamric & Spross, 1989). Although these roles have many times been seen as roles belonging to CNSs, these roles or functions are appropriate for all APNs. NONPF (1995) specified that these four roles were part of the professional role of NPs. Research-based practice is one characteristic that has overwhelmingly been acknowledged as a key characteristic of APNs. Each of these roles will be addressed in subsequent chapters.

The AACN through a consensus building process, formulated curric-

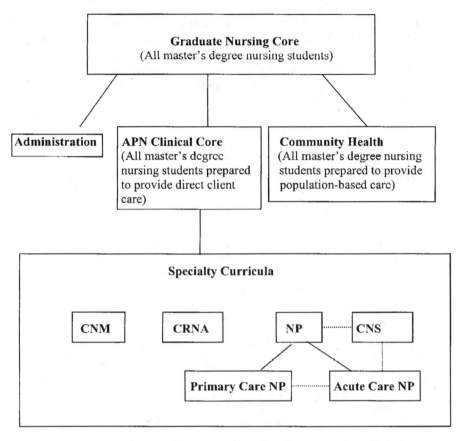

FIGURE 1.1   The AACN conception of graduate nursing education.

Note: From *The essentials of master's education for advanced practice nursing,* by American Association of Colleges of Nursing, 1997, p. 5. Copyright 1997 by the author. Reprinted with permission of the author.

ular elements for graduate advanced practice nursing education. Figure 1.1 depicts the AACN conception of graduate nursing education. Table 1.1 presents the content to be included in the graduate core curriculum and the advanced practice nursing core curriculum.

The core clinical content focuses on advanced health/physical assessment, advanced physiology and pathology, and advanced pharmacology. The AACN notes that this content is of a general nature and that specifics will be needed for students in the various specialty areas. For example, midwifery students would need additional content on assessment of pregnant women and newborn infants. Nurse anesthetist students would require content on anesthetic agents, while psychiatric/mental health students would need additional content on anti-psychotic medications. One area not specified in the AACN core content was nursing therapeutics. With society's increasing use of complementary therapies, it is imperative that APN students receive content about complementary therapies. Many of these therapies have a long history of use in nursing, so APNs should incorporate these therapies into their practice. NONPF (1995) noted that although APN curricula are crowded, strong social pressure exists to include content on complementary therapies.

Although the curriculum and competencies proposed by NONPF (1995) were developed specifically for NP education, the content and competencies have much relevance to the content included in the graduate nursing core. Components of the graduate nursing core, advanced nursing specialty core, and NP specialty are found in Table 1.2. Many commonalities are found between the AACN proposed curriculum and that proposed by NONPF. For example, both see the need for content on research, theory, ethics, health care systems, and cultural diversity. The APN core of NONPF is broader and notes content on clinical decision-making and family theory.

In addition to the content to be included in graduate APN programs, NONPF also proposed domains and competencies for NPs. The five domains are management of client health/illness status, nurse-client relationship, teaching-coaching function, professional role, managing and

TABLE 1.1   Essential Elements of Curriculum for Advanced Practice Nursing Proposed by AACN

Graduate Core Curriculum Elements
   Research
   Policy, Organization, and Financing of Health Care
      Health care policy
      Organization of the health care delivery system
      Health care financing
   Ethics
   Professional Role Development
   Theoretical Foundations of Nursing Practice
   Human Diversity and Social Issues
Advanced Practice Core Elements
   Advanced Health/Physical Assessment
   Advanced Physiology and Pathology
   Advanced Pharmacology

Note: From *The essentials of master's education for advanced practice nursing,* by American Association of Colleges of Nursing, 1997, p. 5.

TABLE 1.2   Components of Nurse Practitioner Education as Proposed by NONPF

Graduate Nursing Core
   Research
   Health Policy
   Nursing and Health-Related Theory
   Organizational Theory
   Ethics
   Cultural Diversity
   Community-based Care
   Health Care Economics
   Health Care Delivery Systems
   Managed Care
Advanced Nursing Practice Core
   Health Assessment
   Pharmacology
   Pathophysiology
   Clinical Decision-making
   Health Promotion/Disease Prevention
   Community-based Practice
   Role
   Family Theory
Nurse Practitioner Specialty
   Specialty Management
   Clinical Practice
   Specialty Role

Source: Adapted from *Advanced nursing practice: Curriculum guidelines and program standards for nurse practitioner education,* National Organization for Nurse Practitioner Faculties, 1995, p. 44.

negotiating health care delivery systems, and monitoring and ensuring the quality of health care practice. These are based on work by Brykczynski (1989), Benner (1984), and Fenton (1985). Specific competencies are specified for each domain. As can be noted, these domains convey that being an APN requires a broad range of knowledge and expertise.

The American Nurses Association has developed practice standards for APNs (ANA, 1996). It is the expectation that APNs will also meet the practice standards contained in the *Standards of Clinical Nursing Practice* (ANA, 1991). Many of the standards relate to content included as essential for APN education by AACN (1997) and NONPF (1995). Table 1.3 contains the focus areas of the standards.

One ANA standard relates to health promotion and health maintenance. Nurses have traditionally espoused health promotion as being a key characteristic of the professional practice of nursing. Health promotion, whether it be for persons who have no specific illness or for persons who have chronic health problems, is critical in our current society. Implementation of care that focuses on health promotion has been shown to be cost effective (Safriet, 1992). Longworth (1993) noted that NPs were consistently more thorough in assessing risk factors for disease and in including health screening in their assessments than were attending staff.

Ethics is another area for an ANA standard for APNs. In addition to issues related to confidentiality and relationships, APNs will provide support to patients and families in making decisions about ethical issues related to treatment decisions. Although ethical issues appear to be more prominent in tertiary care settings, issues such as abuse and neglect are present in all settings. APNs will be called upon to assist staff in resolving ethical dilemmas.

The increasing complexity of care and the provision of care in multiple settings requires that APNs collaborate with other health profes-

TABLE 1.3 Topics of ANA Standards of Practice for Advanced Practice Registered Nurses

Standards of Care
    Assessment
    Diagnosis
    Outcome Identification
    Planning of Care
    Implementation of Care
        Case management
            Consultation
            Health promotion, Health maintenance, and health teaching
            Prescription authority and treatment
            Referral
    Evaluation
Standards of Professional Performance
    Quality of Care
    Self-Evaluation
    Education
    Leadership
    Ethics
    Collaboration
    Research

Source: Adapted from *Scope and standards of advanced practice registered nursing,* American Nurses Association, 1996, pp. 10–11.

sionals. Collaboration is an ANA standard of care. Functioning on inter-disciplinary teams or working in collaboration with other health professionals requires APNs to be able to identify nursing's contributions to patient outcomes. APNs also collaborate with patients and their families in planning care and making decisions about the most acceptable treatments.

As can be noted in the above content about APNs, their educational preparation, and the expectations of the work sites, it can be questioned whether APNs can be prepared in the usual 2-year master's program. This has prompted discussions about whether it would be more appropriate to have APNs prepared in Doctor of Nursing Science (DNSc) programs. One school, Rush University, awards a Nursing Doctorate (ND) degree to students completing NP programs. This is an area requiring further discussion.

Titles, Licensure, and Certification Issues

As noted earlier, discussion has been devoted to the merger of the APN and CNS roles. Although some discussion about merging these two roles continues, primarily because CNS are moving into primary care practice sites and NPs are practicing in tertiary care sites, the debate appears to have lessened. What is clear is that it is essential for nursing to put forward a description of APNs that is applicable to the CNS, NP, CRNA, and nurse-midwife. Great strides have been made in this arena, as demonstrated by the curricular efforts.

Second-level licensure has been proposed by the Association of States' Boards of Nursing. The concern of the State Boards was their societal responsibility for safe practice of nursing. Because such diversity in certification exists, this did not appear to be a means that could be used to ensure the public about the preparation and skills of APNs. Second-level licensure was opposed by the American Nurses' Association. One objection was that no other profession had two levels of licensure. Legally, there was concern that an APN could be sued for breach of practice at two levels.

Since the early 1980s APNs have, of necessity, been active in federal and state politics in order to legalize their scope of practice. Involvement at both levels is necessary since state legislatures are charged with protecting the health and interests of their residents by the regulation of professional practice. Complex political initiatives in each state are required to have APN laws written, lobbied, passed, and enacted through regulations. Legislative actions, at both federal and state levels, have made it possible for APNs to legally practice in new ways. The profession owes a debt of gratitude to the nurses who have had the fortitude to persevere against powerful opponents to provide advanced practice nursing with its legal foundation. In many states, the laws to legitimize APN prescriptive privileges and third-party reimbursement have been added to pharmacy and insurance statutes; in such cases, non-nursing regulatory boards are given jurisdiction over nursing practice (Pearson, 1998). A patchwork of confusing laws and regulations now exists across the country regarding advanced practice nursing. The great variation between the state laws and regulations causes confusion, adds expense, and creates multiple regulatory barriers to APN practice. Particularly impacted are nurses who move from one state to another, or who practice near state borders, thus requiring multiple state licenses.

There are two approaches to legalizing APN practice in state law. One is the more typical approach that has been used in some states in which clauses to existing laws have been added that define APNs as legal prescribers of medications in the state or require insurance companies to reimburse for APN services. A second, less common approach, has been for states to revise their nurse practice act and thus bring together all laws and regulations pertaining to APNs into a single coherent document. Without this comprehensive approach of rewriting state practice acts, APNs are not defined or given title protection under the law (Safriet, 1994). The Pew Commission (1995) criticized existing regulation of the nursing profession and urges states to standardize the statutes related to APNs. In 1997 the National Council of State Boards of Nursing (NCSBN) proposed a multistate mutual recognition model to create more reciprocity for nurses between states and thus to ease the regulatory barriers of interstate practice. Their proposal remains under debate.

Credentialing

In addition to state laws, APNs also encounter other regulatory systems to which they must be accountable, specifically, professional certification organizations, and health care organization credentialling bodies. National APN certification is increasingly required by state laws (generally for prescribing privileges and reimbursement), and is frequently stated as a requirement for employment by facilities hiring APNs. Specific criteria regarding the APN program of studies must be verified before APN graduates can sit for certification examinations. Other criteria related to continuing education and active practice must be met periodically to maintain active APN certification status. It is vital that APNs carefully keep detailed records of basic, graduate, and continuing nursing education throughout their careers, since they are frequently required to produce proof of their preparation to maintain their right to practice at an advanced level.

Other entities may also request APNs to produce documented proof of their legitimacy to practice, a process generally termed credentialling. In order to obtain provider numbers and thus be reimbursed by insurers and governmental payers, APNs undergo credentialling by each third-party reimbursement payer (i.e. Medicare, managed care organizations, private insurers). This process is laborious, as the credentialling process has not been centralized.

The final credentialling process for APNs is carried out by health care organizations in order to appoint APNs to their professional staff. Obtaining staff privileges through being appointed to health care organization professional staff allows APNs to write orders and discharge patients. The specific scope of practice activities is delineated in the credentialling process. For example, CNSs may be credentialled to perform selected invasive procedures; pediatric nurse practitioners may be permitted to examine and discharge infants from a newborn nursery. The criteria and institutional credentialling processes are reviewed by accreditors such as the Joint Commission for Accreditation of Healthcare Organizations (JCAHO). This review may force facilities to change their rules, for example, requiring physician co-signatures on pre-operative physical examinations and thus require APN supervision of this generally independent activity.

CONCLUSION

Advanced practice nurses have made significant contributions to quality health care, particularly for vulnerable populations. Many (Aiken, 1995; Pew Health Professions Commission, 1994b), have noted that if all Americans are to receive quality, cost-effective health care, it is critical that greater use be made of APNs. A bright future awaits nursing and

APNs in the new millennium. Their advanced knowledge and skills, both in nursing and related fields, provide APNs with the capabilities of making valuable contributions to the current health care system and in assuming leadership roles in developing new practice sites or innovative systems of care that will enhance the quality of health care. As America becomes more diverse, APNs will play a key role in ensuring that culturally competent care is delivered.

Although the content in this chapter has focused on APNs in the United States, it is encouraging to see the continuing development of this role in other countries. Clinical specialization in nursing has existed in many countries for centuries. However, in other countries, specialization and use of APNs are only beginning (Nelson-Conley, 1990; Wang, Yen, & Snyder, 1995). Nurses can do much by sharing past experiences, providing support to nurses trying to advance the status of nursing in their countries, and overall, by keeping alive the ideal of nursing's quest to provide quality care for all persons.

REFERENCES

Aiken, L. H. (1995). Transformation of the nursing workforce. *Nursing Outlook, 43,* 201–209.

American Association of Colleges of Nursing. (1997). *The essentials of master's education for advanced practice nursing.* Washington, DC: Author.

American Association of Colleges of Nursing. (1998). *1997–1998 enrollment and graduations in baccalaureate and graduate in nursing.* Washington, DC: Author.

American Association of Nurse Anesthetists. (1992). Qualifications and capabilities of the certified registered nurse anesthetist. *Professional Practice Manual for the Certified Registered Nurse Anesthetist.* Park Ridge, IL: Author.

American Association of Nurse Anesthetists. (1996). Scope and standards for nurse anesthesia practice. *Professional practice manual for the Certified Registered Nurse Anesthetist.* Park Ridge, IL: Author.

American Association of Nurse Anesthetists. (1998, June). 75% of Medicare patients say HCFA is right!. *Newsbulletin, 52*(6), 7.

American College of Nurse-Midwives. (1989). *Philosophy of the American College of Nurse-Midwives* (Position Statement). Washington, DC: Author.

American College of Nurse-Midwives. (1997b). *Definition of a certified nurse-midwife* (Position Statement). Washington, DC: Author.

American College of Nurse-Midwives. (1997c). *Definition of midwifery practice* (Position Statement). Washington, DC: Author.

American College of Nurse-Midwives. (1997a). *The core competencies for basic midwifery practice* (Position Statement). Washington, DC: Author.

American Nurses Association. (1991). *Standards of clinical nursing practice.* Washington, DC: Author.

American Nurses Association. (1995). *Nursing social policy statement.* Washington, DC: Author.

American Nurses Association. (1996). *Scope and standards of advanced practice nursing.* Washington, DC: Author.

Bankert, M. (1989). *Watchful care: A history of America's nurse anesthetists.* New York: Continuum.

Benner, P. E. (1984). *From novice to expert: Excellence and power in clinical nursing practice.* Menlo Park, CA: Addison-Wesley.

Blanchette, H. (1995). Comparison of obstetric outcome of a primary-care access clinic staffed by certified nurse-midwives and a private practice group of obstetricians in the same community. *American Journal of Obstetrics and Gynecology, 172,* 1864–1871.

Brykczynski, K. A. (1989). An interpretive study describing the clinical judgment of nurse practitioners. *Scholarly Inquiry for Nursing Practice: An Interpretive Journal, 3*(2), 113–120.

Cronenwett, L. R. (1995). Molding the future of advanced practice nursing. *Nursing Outlook, 43,* 112–118.

Elder, R. G., & Bullough, B. (1990). Nurse practitioners and clinical nurse specialists: Are the roles merging? *Clinical Nurse Specialist, 4,* 78–84.

Fenton, M. V. (1985). Identifying competencies of clinical nurse specialists. *Journal of Nursing Administration, 15*(12), 31–37.

Fenton, M. V., & Brykczynski, K. A. (1993). Qualitative distinctions and similarities in the practice of clinical nurse specialists and nurse practitioners. *Journal of Professional Nursing, 9,* 313–326.

Forbes, K., Rafson, J., Spross, J. A., & Kozlowski, D. (1990). Clinical nurse specialist and nurse practitioner core curricula survey results. *Nurse Practitioner, 15,* 45–48.

Ford, L. C. (1979). A nurse for all setting: The nurse practitioner. *Nursing Outlook, 27*(8), 516–521.

Ford, L. C., & Silver, H. K. (1967). The expanded role of the nurse in child care. *Nursing Outlook, 15*(9), 43–45.

Hamric, A. B., & Spross, J. A. (1989). *The clinical nurse specialist in theory and practice.* Philadelphia: Saunders.

Jordan, L. (1994). Qualifications and capabilities of the certified registered nurse anesthetist. In S. Foster & L. Jordan (Ed.), *Professional aspects of nurse anesthesia practice* (pp. 3–10). Philadelphia: F.A. Davis.

Kalisch, P. A., & Kalisch, B. J. (1986). *The advance of American nursing.* Boston: Little, Brown.

Kitzman, H. J. (1983). The CNS and nurse practitioner. In A. B. Hamric & J. Spross (Eds.), *The clinical nurse specialist in theory and practice* (pp. 275–290). New York: Grune & Stratton.

Long, K. A. (1994). Master's degree nursing education and health care reform: Preparing for the future. *Journal of Professional Nursing, 10,* 71–76.

Longworth, J. D. (1993, June). RNs will satisfy demand for quality of care. *American Nurse,* 8.

MacDorman, M. F., & Singh, G. K. (1998). Midwifery care, social and medical risk factors, and birth outcomes in the USA. *Journal of Epidemiology & Community Health, 52,* 310–317.

National League for Nursing. (1997). *Nursing data source.* New York: Author.

National Organization of Nurse Practitioner Faculties. (1995). *Advanced nursing practice: Curriculum guidelines and program standards for nurse practitioner education.* Washington, DC: Author.

Naylor, M., Brooten, D., Jones, R., Lavizzo-Mourey, R., Mezey, M., & Pauly, M. (1994). Comprehensive discharge planning for hospitalized elderly: A randomized clinical trial. *Annals of Internal Medicine, 120,* 999–1006.

Neidlinger, S. H., Scroggins, K., & Kennedy, L. M. (1987). Cost evaluation of discharge planning for hospitalized elderly. *Nursing Economics, 5,* 225–230.

Nelson-Conley, C. L. (1990). Role development of the clinical nurse specialist within the Indian health service. *Clinical Health Specialist, 4*(3), 142–146.

Page, N. E., & Arena, D. M. (1994). Rethinking the merger of the clinical nurse specialist and the nurse practitioner roles. *Image: Journal of Nursing Scholarship, 26,* 315–318.

Pearson, L. (1998). Annual update of how each state stands on legislative issues affecting advanced nursing practice. *The Nurse Practitioner, 23*(1), 14–16, 19–20, 25–26.

Pew Health Professions Commission. (1994a). *Nurse practitioners: Doubling the graduates by the year 2000.* San Francisco: University of California, Center for the Health Professions.

Pew Health Professions Commission. (1994b). *Primary care workforce 2000: Federal policy paper.* San Francisco: University of California, Center for the Health Professions.

Pew Health Professions Commission. (1995). Critical challenges: Revitalizing the health professions for the twenty-first century. *The third report of the Pew Health Professions Commission.* Washington, DC: Author.

Rasch, F. R., & Frauman, A. C. (1996). Advanced practice in nursing: Conceptual issues. *Journal of Professional Nursing, 12,* 141–146.

Redekopp, M. A. (1997). Clinical nurse specialist role confusion: The need for identity. *Clinical Nurse Specialist, 11*(2), 87–91.

Reiter, F. (1966). The nurse-clinician. *American Journal of Nursing, 66,* 274–280.

Rosenblatt, R. A., Dobie, S. A., Hart, L. G., Schneeweiss, R., Gould, D., Raine, T. R., Benedetti, T. J., Pirani, M. J., & Perrin, E. B. (1997). Interspecialty differences in the obstetric care of low-risk women. *American Journal of Public Health, 87,* 344–351.

Safriet, B. (1992). Health care dollars and regulatory sense: The role of advanced practice nursing. *Yale Journal of Regulation, 9,* 417–487.

Safriet, B. (1994). Impediments to progress in health care workforce policy: License and practice laws. *Inquiry, 31,* 310–317.

Varney, H. (1997). *Varney's midwifery.* (3rd ed.). Sudbury, MA: Jones and Bartlett.

Ventura, S. J., Martin, J. A., Curtin, C. S., & Matthewa, T. J. (1998). Report of final natality statistics, 1996. *Monthly vital statistics report* (Vol. 46, suppl. p. 17). Hyattsville, MD: National Center for Health Statistics.

Vollman, K. M., & Stewart, K. H. (1996). Can we afford NOT to have clinical nurse specialists? *AACN Clinical Issues, 7,* 315–323.

Wang, J., Yen, M., & Snyder, M. (1995). Constraints and perspectives of advanced practice nursing in Taiwan, Republic of China. *Clinical Nurse Specialist, 9,* 252–255.

Wells, N., Erickson, S., & Spinella, J. (1996). Role transition: From clinical nurse specialist to clinical specialist/case manager. *Journal of Nursing Administration, 26*(11), 23–28.

Chapter 2

ADVANCED PRACTICE WITHIN A NURSING PARADIGM

Mariah Snyder PhD, RN, FAAN

The most important word in the title of Advanced Practice Nurse (APN) is the last one: nurse. Advanced education enables nurses to expand their knowledge base and expertise of nursing so that their practice differs not only from that of nurses with associate or baccalaureate degrees but also from that of other health professionals, particularly physicians. Nurses often underestimate the profound positive effect that their care can have on improving patient outcomes (Lang & Marek, 1992). Nightingale, in *Notes on Nursing* (1959/1992) noted that persons in her day often thought of nursing as signifying "little more than the administration of medicines and the application of poultices" (p.6). Efforts are still necessary to convey the full scope of nursing practice to other professionals and to the public so that nursing's contributions to positive health outcomes are understood, valued, and reimbursed. So often the media has focused s on the physical assessment skills and prescriptive privileges rather than on the distinctive skills and expertise related to nursing that characterize APN practice.

WHAT IS NURSING?

Definitions of Nursing

For many years the nursing profession has sought to define what constitutes nursing and to identify its scope of practice. It is critical for APNs and those aspiring to this role to have a clear understanding of what constitutes nursing so that in interdisciplinary and other interactions they are able to provide a clear understanding of nursing's unique contributions to health care outcomes. Several of the numerous definitions of nursing that have been put forth over the years will be examined.

Florence Nightingale formulated one of the earliest definitions of nursing. Nightingale (1859\1992) defined nursing as having charge of the personal health of a person. The aim of nursing care, according to Nightingale, is to put the patient in the best possible condition so that nature can act upon the person. *Notes on Nursing,* although written almost 150 years ago, speaks to the substantive basis of nursing. Not only does Nightingale elaborate on interventions nurses can employ, but she also underscores the necessity of thorough assessments before planning nursing care. Reading of *Notes on Nursing* should be part of APN curricula.

In Virginia Henderson's (1966) definition of nursing, emphasis is placed on the nurse collaborating with the patient to enhance the patient's health status. Henderson defined nursing as

> assisting the individual, sick or well, in the performance of those activities contributing to health or its recovery (or to a peaceful death) that he would perform unaided if he had the necessary strength, will, or knowledge. And to do this in such a way as to help him gain independence as soon as possible. (p. 15).

Henderson's definition contains many elements that constitute the substantive nature of nursing. Health promotion is a key component of her definition. In addition, the caring aspects of nursing are emphasized. Not all patients will recover from their diseases or injuries. It is the nurse's role to assist patients to achieve the goals the patient has established. Myss (1996) noted in curing modalities, the patient is passive. Conversely, the patient must take an active role to be healed. APNs can play a key role in assisting patients in their healing process. APNs are able to bring additional expertise to interactions with patients and to perform holistic health assessments. Henderson stresses helping the patient gain independence. Independence is truly a Western belief and may not be a value in all cultures. Thus, it is important for the nurse to ascertain the personal values of each patient, and independence may not be one of his/her preferences.

Nojima (1989), a Japanese nursing theorist, defined nursing practice as:

> A human activity carried out by nurses to help individuals organize their health conditions so that they are able to live optimally and realize their potential. (p.6–7)

In her definition, the focus is on a person's quality of life. The partnership between the nurse and the patient is evident in Nojima's definition of nursing.

The American Nurses Association (ANA) has defined nursing as "The diagnosis and treatment of human responses to actual or potential health problems" (1995, p. 6). Persons and their responses to health problems, rather than specific illnesses, are highlighted in the brief definition proposed by the ANA. This focus serves to differentiate nursing from medicine. Despite the frequent reference to the ANA definition of nursing, many APNs have had encountered difficulty in working from a nursing model. They have been forced to launch their practice within the medical model. Although it is important to know the cause of a person's pain or stress, much of nursing care remains the same, despite the etiology. It has been encouraging to see the Agency for Health Care Policy and Research (AHCPR) consider problems or responses, rather than disease entities, as the focus of practice guidelines. For example, practice guidelines have been redeveloped for decubitus ulcers and acute pain.

Scope of Practice

Gaining more knowledge about the substantive basis of nursing is an essential component of APN education.. Numerous initiatives have undertaken to identify, describe, and classify the phenomena of concern to nurses. The findings from these explorations have helped nurses gain an understanding about the scope of nursing practice. A number of initiatives have been carried out to delineate the substantive basis of nursing. Nursing diagnoses and human responses, two of the initiatives, will be discussed.

Nursing diagnoses

Nursing diagnoses are one strategy nurses have used to describe phenomena for which nurses provide care. Since the First Nursing Diagnosis Conference in 1973, nurses within the North American Nursing Diagnosis Association (NANDA) have worked to identify, describe, and validate patient problems/concerns that fall within the domain of nursing. Currently, over 100 diagnoses have been approved, it is projected that eventually there will be over 300 diagnoses (Craft-Rosenberg & Delaney, 1997). Continued efforts are necessary to identify and validate new diagnoses and to revise existing diagnoses. APNs have and can continue to provide leadership in the nursing diagnosis movement.

NANDA diagnoses are grouped under nine patterns: exchanging, communicating, relating, valuing, choosing, moving, perceiving, knowing, and feeling. According to Newman (1984), it is important for nurses to determine changes in a patient's patterns. In approaching assessment in this manner, the focus is the whole rather than specific diagnoses.

Nursing diagnoses have been widely accepted not only in the United States, but also internationally (Coler, da Nobrega, de Almeida Peres, & de Farias, 1991; Snyder, 1989). Nursing diagnoses are the first effort to develop a common language for nursing phenomena. Despite numerous criticisms of nursing diagnoses, use of diagnoses has assisted nurses in focusing on those aspects of care for which nursing interventions can be institutions and nurse-sensitive outcomes can be determined. APNs needs to be familiar with both nursing and medical diagnoses.

In addition to establishing a common language for nursing diagnoses, the International Council of Nurses is working on identifying and classifying nursing interventions and outcomes (International Council of Nurses Project, 1997). In the United States, a number of projects to identify and classify nursing interventions have been initiated. The National Intervention Classification (NIC) has identified and classified over 433 interventions (McCloskey & Bulechek, 1996). Likewise, a project to identify nursing outcomes is being conducted at the University of Iowa (Johnson, 1997).

Human responses

The American Nurses Association has delineated phenomena of concern to nursing (ANA, 1995). The identified phenomena were not meant to be exhaustive, but rather to be exemplars of the types of concerns that fall

TABLE 2.1   Human Responses That are the Focus for Nursing Intervention

Care and self-care processes
Physiological and psychological processes—such as rest, sleep, respiration,
    circulation, reproduction, nutrition, elimination, sexuality, and communication
Physical and emotional comfort, discomfort, and pain
Emotions related to experiences of birth, health, illness, and death
Meanings ascribed to health and illness
Decision-and choice-making abilities
Perceptual orientations such as self-image and control over one's body
Relationships, role performance, and change processes within relationships
Social policies and their effects on the health of individuals, families, and
    communities

Note. From *Nursing's Social Policy Statement* (p. 8), by American Nurses Association, 1995, Washington, DC: American Nurses Publishing. Copyright 1995 by the Association. Reprinted with permission.

within the purview of nursing. Human responses identified by ANA are found in Table 2.1.

As with nursing diagnoses, these identified human responses assist APNs to focus on the health concerns for which nursing care is primary in producing positive patient outcomes. Therapeutics for managing the responses or assisting the person to manage transcend medical entities. For example, despite various etiologies for sleep problems, nursing interventions, such as massage and music therapy, can be used to manage sleep problems. Viewing nursing from the perspective of human responses helps nurses to organize content from a nursing perspective.

THE ART AND SCIENCE OF NURSING

The Art of Nursing

The art of nursing is integrally tied to the caring aspect of nursing. Moore (1992), a clinical psychologist, stated that care is what a nurse does. For many years, nursing was defined as being an art and a science. As nursing began to give more attention to establishing a scientific basis for practice and become accepted within the scientific community, the art or caring aspect of nursing received less attention. In practice settings, nurses gave increasing attention to the high technology used in the care of patients with complex health problems. Currently, the public has indicated that they value caring interventions such as massage, touch, and aromatherapy. A number of reasons that persons seek complementary therapies have been proposed: they wish to be treated as a whole person and not just a disease; they desire better communication with the health professional; they wish to be active participants in their care; they desire that the treatment not be worse than the disease; and they feel that Western health care does not meet all of their needs. Therefore, it is important that APNs consider how they can include the art of nursing, which includes traditional nursing interventions into their practice. Efforts are needed to develop a scientific basis for these caring interventions. Chapter 8 provides an overview of complementary therapies.

Caring is a critical element of nursing practice. Leininger (1990), Watson (1988), and Gadow (1980) have put forth definitions of caring. Watson defined the art of caring as:

> A human activity consisting of the following: a nurse consciously, by means of certain signs, passes on to others feelings he or she has lived through, realized, or learned; others are united to these feelings and also experience them. (p. 68)

Newman, Sime, and Corcoran-Perry (1991) noted that the focus of nursing is "caring in the human health experience" (p. 3). Caring has been identified by NONPF as a characteristic of APNs.

Caring requires that a nurse be competent in assessing and intervening. Benner (1988) noted that a caring attitude was not sufficient to make an action a caring practice. The practice must be implemented in an excellent manner in order to be viewed as caring. Caring and the art of nursing convey very similar meanings. Caring nurses seek the scientific basis for their practice and continue to update their expertise and knowledge. APNs possess the knowledge and ability to critique research about specific therapies and determine their applicability to specific patient populations.

Science of nursing

Nursing is characterized by both art and science. Significant progress has been made in developing the knowledge base that underlies nursing practice. However, much additional research is needed before APNs will have a sound scientific basis that will assist them in choosing specific interventions for a patient or population. The clinical guidelines developed by the Agency on Health Care Policy and Research are an example of work that has and continues to be done in identifying "best practices" based on research findings. APNs have a key role in assisting nurses to review research and develop clinical guidelines that incorporate the existing knowledge base.

THEORETICAL/CONCEPTUAL MODELS

During the past 50 years, nursing has given considerable attention to theoretical and conceptual models. This attention has served to differentiate nursing from other disciplines (Engebretson, 1997). Nursing theories are not, however, new in nursing. Nightingale (1859/1992) elaborated the relationship of the environment to health and well-being. Numerous theoretical and conceptual models exist.

What relevance do nursing theories have to practice? Cannot nurses merely practice nursing? Meleis (1985) noted that a theory articulates and communicates a mental image of a certain order that exists in the world. This image includes the components of that order and the relationship(s) among those components. All nurses have a model or perspective that guides their practice. This model may be identical to one of the publicized nursing theories, or it may be based on a theoretical perspective from another discipline. In some instances, eclectic models are used in which nurses combine elements from established nursing theories or theories from other disciplines. New nursing theories continue to be developed. Of particular importance is the delineation of nursing theories that incorporate various cultural perspectives, as to date the Western philosophical perspective has pervaded many of the existing theories.

Discussion has ensued on whether one grand nursing theory for nursing is needed. Would the existence of a grand or meta-theory be advantageous to the progression of the profession and discipline? Riehl-Sisca (1989) stated that nursing has benefited from having a multiplicity of theories. The wide range of perspectives elaborated in these theories has assisted nurses to more clearly define the nature of the discipline and profession, to evaluate various approaches that can be employed in practice, and to respect diversity as a positive element. Marriner-Tomey (1994) identified seven theorists who have developed grand theories or conceptual frameworks for nursing: Johnson, King, Levine, Neuman, Orem, Rogers, and Roy. Numerous other nurses have developed midrange theories or conceptual frameworks that have served as a basis for research and practice.

More recently, nurses have turned their attention to midrange theories. Midrange theories, according to Olson and Hanchett (1997), focus on a limited number of variables. Midrange theories also are more amenable to empirical testing than are grand theories, as they are more concrete and limited in scope. Examples of midrange theories include empathy (Olson & Hanchett, 1997), uncertainty in illness (Mishel,1990), resilience (Polk, 1997), mastery (Younger, 1991), self-transcendence (Reed, 1991), caring (Swanson, 1991, and illness trajectory (Wiener & Dodd, 1993).

Many nurses give little thought to the tenets that guide their practice; however, these philosophical underpinnings have a profound impact on the nature and scope of their practice. Nurses have an ethical responsibility to practice nursing with a consciously defined approach to care. The theoretical or conceptual model used by a nurse provides the basis for making the complex decisions that are crucial in the delivery of good nursing care. Smith (1995) stated

> The core of advanced practice nursing lies within nursing's disciplinary perspective on human-environment and caring interrelationships that facilitate health and healing. This core is delineated specifically in the philosophic and theoretic foundations of nursing. (p. 3)

Thus, nursing theory is an important component of APN education.

Nursing is a practice discipline, and theories achieve importance in relation to their impact on nursing care. Only recently have attempts been made to relate nursing theories to practice and to begin to test these theories. However, only minimal testing of these theories in practice settings has occurred. The numerous theoretical nursing studies, particularly studies examining the efficacy of nursing interventions, is an indication of the seemingly separation of theories and practice that has characterized much of nursing practice.

The theoretical or conceptual framework that an APN selects and uses has a major impact on the patient assessments that are made and the nature of interventions that are chosen to achieve patient outcomes. Gordon (1987) and Johnson (1989) have noted the profound impact a nurse's theoretical perspective can have on nursing practice. Gordon (1987) stated:

> One's conceptual perspective on clients and on nursing's goals strongly determines what kinds of things one assesses. Everyone has a perspective, whether in conscious awareness or not. Problems can arise if the perspective "in the head" is inconsistent with the actions taken during assessment. Information collection has to be logically related to one's view of nursing. (p. 69)

A conceptual model provides the practitioner with a general perspective or a mind set of what is important to observe and which, in turn, provides the bases for making nursing diagnoses and selecting nursing interventions.

INCORPORATING NURSING INTO ADVANCED PRACTICE NURSING

APNs provide health care to many populations and in many settings. Opportunities exist for APNs to make major contributions to the advancement of the substantive basis of nursing. APNs, by focusing on the nursing elements of health care, have the opportunity to demonstrate to the public and to policymaking bodies the unique and significant contributions that nursing has to health outcomes. Using the nursing rather than the medical model as the focus of practice results in advanced practice nursing presenting the public with a distinct model of care rather than a substitutive model (replacing physicians). Activities that have traditionally been a part of medicine may be carried out by APNs, but the performance of these activities by an APN need to be translated into the realm of nursing. For example, Mitchell and Irvin (1977) noted that neuroscience nurses may do the same neurological assessment as physicians. Nurses use the information obtained in a different manner than do physicians: they use it to monitor the patient's condition and to select nursing interventions.

Guaranteeing that APNs view the provision of health care from a nursing perspective has implications for graduate curricula. Huch (1995) proposed weaving content on nursing theories throughout the APN curriculum. Not only is content needed, but students also needs assistance in utilizing this theoretical content in their practice. Faculty and preceptors who model the application of theory in practice are critical for helping APN students integrate theory into their practice.

REFERENCES

American Nurses Association. (1995). *Nursing: A Social Policy Statement.* Washington, D.C.: Author.

Benner, P. (1988). *Nursing as a caring profession.* Paper presented at the meeting of American Academy of Nursing, Kansas City, MO.

Coler, M. S., de Nobrega, M. M., de Almeida Perse V. L., & deFarias, J. N. (1991). A Brazilian study of two diagnoses in the NANDA human response pattern, Moving: A transcultural comparison. In R. Carroll-Johnson (ed.), *Classification of nursing diagnoses* (pp. 255–256). Philadelphia: Lippincott.

Craft-Rosenberg, M. & Delaney (1997). Nursing diagnosis extension and classification. In M. J. Rantz & P. LeMone (Eds.), *Classification of nursing diagnoses: Proceedings of the 12th conference* (pp. 26–31). Pittsburgh, PA: NANDA.

Engebretson, J. (1997). A multiparadigm approach to nursing. *Advances in Nursing Science, 20*(1), 21–33.

Gadow, S. (1980). Body and self: A dialectic. *The Journal of Medicine and Philosophy, 5,* 172–184.

Gordon, M. (1987). *Nursing Diagnoses.* New York: McGraw-Hill.

Henderson, V. (1966). *Nature of Nursing.* New York: Macmillan.

Huch, M. H. (1995). Nursing science as a basis for advanced practice. *Nursing Science Quarterly, 8*(1), 6–7.

International Council of Nursing. (1997). *The Internatinal Classification for Nursing Practice: A Unifying Framework.* Geneva, Switzerland: Author.

Johnson, D. E. (1959). The nature of a science of nursing. *Nursing Outlook, 7*(4), 198–200.

Johnson, D. E. (1980). The behavioral system model for nursing. In J. P. Riehl & C. Roy (Eds.), *Conceptual models for nursing practice* (2nd ed., pp. 207–216). New York: Appleton-Century-Crofts.

King, I. M. (1971). *Toward a theory of nursing.* New York: Wiley.

Lang, N. M., & Marek, K. D. (1992). Outcomes that reflect clinical practice. In *Patient outcomes research: Examining the effectiveness of nursing practice*

(NIH Publishing No. 93–3411, pp. 27–38). Washington, D.C.: U.S. Department of Health and Human Services.

Leininger, M. (1990). Historic and epistemologic dimensions of care and caring with future directions. In J. Stevenson & T. Tripp-Reimer (Eds.), *Knowledge about care and caring* (pp. 19–31). kansas City, MO: American Academy of Nursing.

Levine, M. (1967). The four conservation principles of nursing. *Nursing Forum, 6*(1), 45–59.

Maas, M. (1997). Nursing-sensitive outcomes classification (NOC): Completing the essential comprehensive languages for nursing. In M. J. Rantz & P. LeMone (Eds.), *Classification of nursing diagnoses: Proceedings of the 12th conference* (pp. 40–47). Pittsburgh, PA: NANDA.

Marriner-Tomey, A. (1993). *Nursing theorists and their work* (3rd ed.). St. Louis, MO: Mosby.

McCloskey, J. C., & Bulecehk, G. M. (Eds.). (1996). *Nursing interventions classification (NIC): Iowa intervention project* (2nd ed.). St. Louis, MO: Mosby.

Meleis, A. I. (1985). *Theoretical nursing: Development and progress.* Philadelphia: Lippincott.

Mishel, M. H. (1990). Reconceptualization of the uncertainty in illness theory. *Image: Journal of Nursing Scholarship, 22,* 256–262.

Mitchell, P. H., & Irvin, N. (1977). Neurological exmaination: Nursing assessment for nursing purposes. *Journal of Neurosurgical Nursing, 9,* 23–27.

Moore, T. (1992). *Care of the soul.* New York: Harper Collins.

Myss, C. (1996). *Anatomy of the spirit.* New York: Three Rivers Press.

Neuman, B. (1974). The Betty Neuman health-care system model: A total person approach to patient problems. In J. P. Riehl & C. Roy (Eds.), *Conceptual models for nursing practice* (pp. 99–114). New York: Appleton-Century-Crofts.

Newman, M. A. (1984). Looking at the whole. *American Journal of Nursing, 84,* 1496–1499.

Newman, M. A., Sime, A. M., & Corcoran-Perry, S. A. (1991). The focus of the discipline of nursing. *Advances in Nursing Science, 14*(1), 1–6.

Nightingale, F. (1992). *Notes on nursing.* Philadelphia: Lippincott. (Originally published 1859).

Nojima, Y. (1989, May). *The structural formula of nursing practice: A bridge to new nursing.* Paper presented at the 19th Quadrennial Congress of the International Congress of Nurses, Seoul, Korea.

Olson, J., & Hanchett, E. (1997). Nurse-expressed empathy, patient outcomes, and development of a middle-range theory. *Image, 29,* 71–76.

Orem, D. E. (1980). *Nursing: Concepts of Practice.* New York: McGraw-Hill.

Polk, L. V. (1997). Toward a middle-range theory of resilience. *Advances in Nursing Science, 19*(3), 1–13.

Reed, P. G. (1991). Toward a nursing theory of self-transcendence: Deductive reformulation using developmental theories. *Advances in Nursing Science, 13*(4), 64–71.

Riehl-Sisca, J. (1989). *Conceptual models for nursing practice.* Norwalk, CT: Appleton & Lange.

Rogers, M. (1970). *An introduction to the theoretical basis of nursing.* Philadelphia: Davis.

Roy, C. (1984). *Introduction to nursing: An adaptation model.* Englewood Cliffs, N.J.: Prentice-Hall.

Smith, M. C. (1995). The core of advanced practice nursing. *Nursing Science Quarterly, 8*(1), 2–3.

Snyder, M. (1989). Nursing diagnoses: Moving nursing forward. *Japanese Journal of Nursing Education, 30,* 807–814.

Swanson, K. M. (1991). Empirical development of a middle-range theory of caring. *Nursing Research, 40,* 161–166.

Watson, J. (1988). *Nursing: Human science and human care: A theory of nursing.* New York: National League for Nursing.

Wiener, C. L., & Dodd, M. J. (1993). Coping amid uncertainty: An illness trajectory. *Scholarly Inquiry in Nursing Practice, 7*(1), 17–30.

Younger, J. B. (1991). A theory of mastery. *Advances in Nursing Science, 14*(1), 76–89.

Chapter 3

PROFESSIONAL ISSUES: LICENSURE AND CERTIFICATION, PRESCRIPTIVE PRIVILEGES, AND REIMBURSEMENT

Michaelene P. Mirr, RN, PhD, CS
Linda Lindeke, PhD, RN, CPNP

Advanced practice nurses (APNs) encounter a variety of professional issues in their practice. Most questions focus on what APNs can or cannot do within the realm of nursing practice. Approximately 60–80% of the primary and preventive care traditionally performed by doctors could be performed by nurses in advanced practice if legislative barriers did not exist (Cassetta, 1993). The shifts in care from acute care to community-based settings has provided new opportunities for nurses in advanced practice. With these opportunities, new issues related to advanced practice have emerged. The focus of this chapter will be on questions related to licensure, certification, prescriptive authority, reimbursement, and clinical privileges. Inherent in these questions is the need for legislative awareness and action on the part of all nurses in advanced practice. The passage of the 1997 Balanced Budget Act and subsequent Health Care Financing Administration Ruling Medicare reimbursement for NP's and CNS's is an excellent example of the importance of an active legislative role.

LICENSURE

Licensure is defined as the "process by which an agency of government grants permission to persons to engage in a given profession or occupation by certifying that those licensed have attained a minimum degree of competency necessary to ensure that the public health, safety and welfare be reasonably protected" (Mirr, 1981, p. 10). Entry-level professional nurses are governed by nurse practice acts passed in each state. As the roles of nurses expanded in the 1970s, many state nurse practice acts were revised to included the added responsibilities nurses assumed. State legislatures chose several methods to provide legal liability for expanded nursing roles. Most states provided for jurisdiction of advanced practice nurses under the nurse practice acts overseen by state boards of nursing. As of 1998, 42 boards of nursing regulated advanced practice (Pearson, 1998).

Licensure, particularly second licensure, is a controversial issue in nursing. Ambiguity that exists regarding consistent qualifications for advanced nursing practice contributes to the movement for second licensure for advanced nursing practice. The National Council of State Boards of Nursing (NCSBN) and the ANA have held opposing viewpoints. The NCSBN states that licensure "is the only regulatory method that bars all others from practicing or representing themselves as APRNs (advanced practice registered nurses)" (Sheets, 1993, p. 9) and provides legitimacy to diagnose and treat illness as well as establish a foundation for direct reimbursement. The ANA argues that no other profession requires multiple licenses to practice one profession (Malone, 1993). For example, an oncologist is not required to have one license to practice as a medical doctor and one license to practice as an oncologist.

Historically, nurse practice acts were created to protect the public from unsafe nursing care. The early acts were written with minimal requirements to enchance enforcement of the status. Two levels of licensure could potentially fragment nursing politically, and would complicate any disciplinary actions that may be needed (Malone, 1993). For example, if an advanced practice nurse is found negligent in advanced practice, would this nurse's professional nursing license also be in jeopardy? Communication between two boards of nursing (basic and APN) related to disciplinary actions would be of great importance.

Licensure is often tied with certification. There have been discussions between credentialing organizations and the National Organization of

Nurse Practitioner Faculties (NONPF) concerning the linkage of educational guidelines with certification or program approval.

Multistate licensure for registered professional nurses has been initiated as increasing numbers of nurses are involved in telehealth activities over state lines. A Multistate Registration Task Force proposed a voluntary system whereby nurses licensed in one state would have authority to practice in states that enter into multistate agreements. The individual would have multistate privileges but would possess only one license. One example is an Interstate Compact (ISC), a legal contract between two or more states that allows nurses to practice in any of the states in the contract agreement. An ISC would be an additional statutory layer above the participating state's Nurse Practice Act (ACNP, 1998b). An advanced practice task force has also been set up to develop an Interstate Contract for advanced practice nurses.

CERTIFICATION

Certification is becoming an increasingly important issue for advanced practice nurses. Certification by a national board is often a requirement for regulatory processes such as prescriptive authority. Certification differs from licensure in that certification is a process by which a nongovernmental agency or association certifies that an individual licensed to practice a profession has met certain predetermined standards specified by that profession for specialty practice. The purpose of certification is to assure various publics that an individual has mastered a body of knowledge and acquired skills in a particular specialty.

Certification in nursing is murky, and equipped with no uniform standard. Many specialty organizations certify nurses with varying educational backgrounds at one general level. The American Nurses' Credentialing Center (ANCC) certifies nurses at various levels with different educational and practice requirements (i.e., gerontological nurse, gerontological nurse practitioner, gerontological clinical nurse specialist). Previous attempts to set up an umbrella certification organization have been unsuccessful. The proliferation of advanced practice programs during the 1990s has added to the concern that educational programs preparing individuals for certification undergo an approval process. The National Council of State Boards of Nursing acknowledged that ANCC certification exams meet their goals verifying that they can be used for regulatory purposes and legal defensibility (ANCC, 1997b).

The ANCC provides certification for the nursing profession which guarantees to the public that a nurse has a certain level of knowledge or skill. The ANCC grew from the ANA Certification Program established in 1973 to an independent center through which ANA would serve as its own credentialing program. Goals of the ANCC include "promoting and enhancing public health by certifying nurses and accrediting organizations using ANA standards of nursing practice, nursing services, and continuing education" (ANCC, 1997a, p. 3).

The ANCC offers certification for clinical nurse specialists in five areas: medical surgical nursing, gerontological nursing, community health nursing, adult psychiatric and mental health nursing, and child and adolescent psychiatric and mental health nursing. The ANCC also certifies nurse practitioners in six clinical areas: adult, family, acute care, school, pediatrics, and gerontology.

Other organizations also offer certification opportunities for nurses. The American Academy of Nurse Practitioners offers certification for adult and family nurse practitioners. Although most specialty organizations provide certification for professional nursing practice, a few offer certification at an advanced practice level. The National Certification Corporation for the Obstetric, Gynecological and Neonatal Nursing Specialties offers certification for the obstetrical/gynecological nurse practitioner and neonatal nurse practitioner. The National Certification Corporation was formerly known as the NAACOG Certification Corporation (NAACOG has been renamed the Association for Women's Health, Obstetrics and Neonatal Nursing) and became an independent certification organization in 1991. Pediatric nurses can also be certified by the National Board of Pediatric Nurse Practitioners and Associates. The Oncology Nursing Society has recently provided certification for advanced nursing practice in oncology.

Prior to 1993, nurses in advanced practice passing the nurse practitioner examinations offered by ANCC were given the title "certified" along with their practitioner specialty, whereas those taking the clinical nurse specialist examination were given the credentials "CS" (Certified Specialist) after their name. Since 1993, all advanced practice nurses passing certification examinations or renewing their certification are given the credential "CS" after their name and professional title (i.e., "Jane Smith, RN, CS"). However, nurse practitioners and clinical specialists still take separate certification examinations.

TABLE 3.1 Sample ANCC Examination Topics

Nurse Practitioner
- Evaluation and promotion of client wellness
- Assessment and management of client illness
- Nurse-client relationships
- Professionalism in advanced nursing practice
- Trends and issues in primary care
- Health policy
- Organizational issues

Clinical Nurse Specialist
- Clinical practice
- Consultation
- Education
- Management
- Research
- Issues and trends

Note: From "Advanced Practice Board Certification Catalog," (pp. 16–22), by American Nurses Credentialing Center, 1998. Washington, DC: Author.

Criteria for Certification

ANCC and AANP require a master's degreee in nursing for nurses to be eligible for certification exams. ANCC criteria for certification as an advanced practice nurse have become more stringent. Nurse practitioners certified by ANCC prior to 1992 were "grandpersoned" in, but must meet recertification criteria for renewal. Eligibility requirements for ANCC certification as a clinical nurse specialist have included a master's degree in nursing since the certification examinations were first implemented.

Current eligibility requirements for certification as a nurse practitioner included possession of an active registered nurse license in the United States or territories, a master's or higher degree in nursing, and preparation as a nurse practitioner in a master's degree program or a formal postgraduate program within a graduate nursing program. Each specialty area may have different requirements. For example, some specialties may have a practice requirement for ANCC recertification. AANP has a practice requirement for family and adult recertification. Eligibility requirements for certification as a clinical nurse specialist include possession of a current active registered nurse license in the United States or territories, a master's degree in nursing, and ability to meet the minimum practice requirement for that clinical specialty.

Guidelines for educational preparation for the specific advanced practice certification examinations are provided in the American Nurses Credentialing Center Advanced Practice Certification Catalog which is updated annually (ANCC, 1997a). Table 3.1 provides general examination topics for ANCC certification examinations. Other organizations, such as the American Academy of Nurse Practitioners, provide annual updates regarding certification.

Advanced practice educational programs may have separate CNS and NP programs, or may offer an integrated advanced practice program within a specialization. Graduates from integrated advanced practice programs have to choose between CNS or designated NP certification exams, because at the present time there are no plans to combine the two.

PRESCRIPTIVE AUTHORITY

One of the biggest obstacles to autonomy in advanced nursing practice is the issue of prescriptive authority. The ability to prescribe medications allows the APN more flexibility in implementing care for clients. Although great strides in legislative efforts have been made in recent years regarding prescriptive authority, the lack of legislative consistency across states has restricted the APN's ability to practice fully within the realm of nursing. Prescriptive authority can be granted in several ways. The use of formularies is a common type of prescriptive authority. APNs are allowed to prescribe drugs that are included in a list (formulary) that has been preapproved by the state regulating board. Another type of prescriptive authority is that of collaborative arrangements between an APN and an affiliated physician, which allows the APN to prescribe. A third type of providing prescriptive authority is recognition of the advanced practice nurses by state statutes as individuals with prescriptive authority (Carson, 1993).

Nurses in advanced practice in some states have had prescriptive authority since the 1970s. The first states to provide legislation granting prescriptive authority were Washington, Oregon, and Alaska. These three states have the least restrictive laws governing prescriptive authority. All states now have some form of statutory prescriptive authority (Pearson, 1999). Eighteen states allow advanced practice nurses to prescribe in-

TABLE 3.2   Advanced Practice Nurse Prescriptive Authority

Independent Prescribing Privileges Including Controlled Substances
AK, AZ, DC, ME, MT, NH, NM, OR, VT, WA, WI

Prescribing Privileges with Physician Involvement Including Controlled Substances
AR, CA, CO, CT, DE, FL, GA, IA, ID, IL, IN, KS, MA, MD, MN, MS, NC, ND, NE, NY, OK, RI, SC, SD, TN, VA, VT, WV, WY

Prescribing Privileges with Physician Involvement Excluding Controlled Substances
AL, HI, KY, LA, MI, MO, NV, OH, TX

Note: From "Annual Update of How Each State Stands on Legislative Issues Affecting Advanced Nursing Practice," by L. Pearson, 1999, *Nurse Practitioner, 24*(1), p. 19. Copyright 1999 by Springhouse Corporation. Reprinted with permission.

dependently including controlled substances. Nineteen states have some degree of physician involvement including controlled substances. Twelve states have some degree of physician collaboration excluding controlled substances. Table 3.2 summarizes prescribing practices in the United States.

Another issue surrounding prescriptive authority is the language used in some regulations and legislation. Some rules and regulations specify "nurse practitioner," excluding clinical nurse specialists, certified nurse-midwives, and certified registered nurse anesthetists. Increasingly, legislation is written to reflect the expanded advanced practice title. Terms that have been used include "midlevel practitioner," "midlevel provider," and "advanced practice nurse." Terms such as "midlevel practitioner" often refer to nurse practitioners, clinical nurse specialists, and physician assistants. Active participation in the political process by professional nursing lobbyists and individual advanced practice nurses has resulted in positive legislative benefits for advanced practice nurses.

APNs can indirectly prescribe medications for patients in states in which APNs do not specifically have legislative authority to prescribe. APNs can request physicians to write prescriptions for the APN's patient. This method is cumbersome and not efficient. Other methods used by APNs to prescribe medications are to call prescriptions into the pharmacy under a physician's name or cosign the physician's prescription pad. Another common practice is the use of protocols mutually agreed upon by the APN and physician (Inglis & Kjervik, 1993).

TABLE 3.3   Inconsistencies Across States Regarding Prescriptive Authority by Advanced Practice Nurses

- statutes or regulations allowing APNs to act and prescribe without MD supervision or collaboration;
- statutes or regulations that limit APN ability by requiring MD supervision such as practice arrangements, protocols, or collaboration;
- statutes or regulations that limit nurse prescriptive authority to certain sites or special community needs;
- limiting prescriptive authority to formularies;
- limiting prescriptive authority by drug schedules;
- limiting prescriptive authority to controlled substances;
- regulations which split prescriptive authority;
- limiting prescriptive authority to physician cosigner;
- statutes or regulations which allow nurses to "order" drugs.

Note: From "Gains and Challenges in Prescriptive Authority" by W. Carson, 1993, *The American Nurse, 25,* pp. 19–20.

Other trends serve to restrict or limit prescriptive practice. These include movement toward joint regulation (joint board with pharmacy, medicine, and nursing); reluctance to "grandperson" in nurses with existing prescriptive authority; ignoring of state boards of nursing's actions by other governmental agencies; restricting drug utilization review boards to pharmacists and physicians; and refusal by pharmaceutical agencies to acknowledge APNs. For example, restriction on prescribing controlled substances limits the prescriptive authority for the APN. Inconsistencies in prescriptive authority for the APN between states contributes to the frustration of APNs' ability to prescribe medications. Table 3.3 summarizes the inconsistencies of legislation among states regarding prescriptive authority (Carson, 1993).

In 1991, the Drug Enforcement Agency (DEA) proposed rules for affiliated practitioners (i.e., nurse practitioners, physician assistants) that would have imposed restrictive regulations for nurses in advanced practice that superseded state laws. The DEA rules did not acknowledge the existing prescriptive regulations in states. Nurses in independent practice would have been affected by the ruling. However the DEA withdrew these proposed rules following a massive protest from the nursing community. A second ruling, entitled "Definition and Registration of Mid-Level Practitioners," was proposed in 1992 (Federal Register, 1992). This new ruling is less restrictive regarding prescriptive writing by nurses in advanced practice. Nurses may apply for and obtain individual DEA registration numbers. DEA registration numbers allow APNs to

dispense controlled substances from schedules II through V as allowed by state law (Inglis & Kjervik, 1993).

Drug Utilization Review Programs mandated by the Omnibus Budget Reconciliation Act of 1990 effective January 1, 1993 were designed to reduce fraud, abuse, overuse, or unnecessary care among physicians, pharmacists, and patients. Currently, no state specifically provides for the inclusion of nurses or other health care members on the review program board. The exclusion of nurses from these boards is of concern, since prescriptive practices by nurses will thus be evaluated by individuals lacking a nursing perspective.

REIMBURSEMENT

Reimbursement for services provided by APNs has been given considerable attention. Federal and state legislation have dictated the level of reimbursement an APN can receive. Moreover, a lag often occurs in the implementation of federal and state rules and policies after legislation has been passed. For example, the 1997 Balanced Budget Act (PL 105-33) provides direct Medicare reimbursement for Nurse Practitioners and Clinical Nurse Specialists. The legislation was passed in 1997 with implementation beginning January 1, 1998. The rules governing this law and written by the Health Care Financing Administration were finalized in November, 1998 (American College of Nurse Practitioners, 1998).

Types of Reimbursement

Many different entities reimburse providers and health systems for care. The payment entities for reimbursement can be grouped as follows:

1. For profit corporations and insurers such as Aetna and Prudential
2. Government payment programs, such as Medicare, Medicaid, Civilian Health and Medical Program of the United States (CHAMPUS)
3. Non-profit corporations, such as Blue Cross/Blue Shield

4. Self-insured corporations or coalitions, such as the Dayton-Hudson Corporation and the Buyers' Health Care Action Group.

These types of health care payers each have reimbursement policies and procedures which differ greatly. They compete and bid for the most favorable service contracts from provider systems and networks. Thus health care finance is volatile, and provider systems are under constant review. There is great variability in the extent to which the various reimbursement entities recognize APNs for reimbursement purposes. Being individually identified through credentialing to obtain reimbursement is essential in order for APNs to have their contributions identified by the above health care payers (Finefrock & Hardy Havens, 1997). Some systems do allow APNs to individually bill for their services under their own name; CHAMPUS, is one example of this practice. Others refuse to reimburse APNs individually, even in states that have had mandated third-party APN reimbursement laws. As Medicare and Medicaid move toward a managed care reimbursement model rather than a fee-for-service model, APNs must be very cognizant of the changes in APN reimbursement policies and procedures (Ferguson, 1996; Mittlestadt, 1998).

Systems of care also have policies and practices that affect APN reimbursement. There are many types of provider systems, such as:

1. Managed care organizations and networks, such as HMOs and PPOs;
2. Private practice, fee-for-service;
3. Home health care and public health agencies; and
4. Specifically funded health care centers, such as community health centers, federal qualified health centers, migrant health clinics, Indian health clinics, and hospitals.

These systems have policies which affect APNs, such as credentialing for reimbursement and hospital privileges, membership on provider panels, and scope of practice parameters. In some instances, federal or state regulations mandate that health care systems identify and specifically reimburse APNs, such as in federally Qualified Health Centers. In more recently developed systems, however, APNs are required to lobby for their place and power within the organization. APNs must be in leadership positions in these provider systems in order to have their contributions to patient outcomes identified and therefore valued by the administration.

Selected Entities and Provider Systems

Medicare

Medicare is a two-part federally funded health care program. Approximately 95% of the nation's elderly are enrolled in Medicare Part A. Part A provides hospital insurance which covers inpatient services, up to 100 days in a skilled nursing facility following hospitalization if needed, and home health care. Although there is no premium required for Part A, a cost-sharing component exists. Cost sharing consists of an annual deductible as well as a percentage of the payment. Medicare does not cover eye examinations, preventive services, medications, or long-term nursing care (ANA, 1993). Part B is a supplementary medical insurance (SMI) that requires a nominal monthly premium from the recipient. Part B pays for physician visits, services and supplies, outpatient services, and home health care (ANA, 1993).

Medicare is oriented to acute care and predominantly serves the elderly. Prior to 1997, only limited reimbursement for nurse practitioners existed. The Omnibus Budget Reconciliation Act (OBRA) of 1989 provides coverage of nurse practitioner services rendered to long-term care facilities. The Omnibus Reconciliation Act of 1990 revised Medicare laws to cover services to nursing home residents provided by advanced practice nurses (nurse practitioners and clinical nurse specialists) in rural areas.

The 1997 Balanced Budget Act (PL 105-33) enacted on August 5, 1997 allows reimbursement of services provided by nurse practitioners and clinical nurse specialists if the services are reimbursable when provided by a physician and the services are within the scope of practice. Therefore, the geographical and setting restrictions of previous legislation were removed. The rules for the legislation written by the Health Care Financing Administration (HCFA) interpret the law positively for NPs and CNSs.

The new law removed the restriction on the type of area and setting in which NPs receive direct Medicare payments. The lifting of the prior restrictions allows NPs and CNSs to submit fees for services rendered in a variety of settings: hospital, skilled nursing facility, nursing home, comprehensive outpatient rehabilitation facility (CORF), community mental health center (CMHC), rural health center (RHC) or federally qualified health center (FQHC).

Payments to NPs and CNSs are "80% of the lesser of either the actual charge or 85% of the physician fee schedule amount" (ACNP, 1998a, p. 2). To avoid double-billing, NPs and CNSs are required to submit their own billing number (UPIN). If the APN is a member of a group practice, the group practice PIN number is used on one line, and the advanced practice nurse's UPIN on another line of the Medicare form. The NP-UPIN will also provide additional information to assess the quality and volume of services performed by NPs (ACNP, 1998a).

Prior to 1997, NPs or CNSs not working in a rural setting or skilled nursing facility submitted payment for services rendered under a provision called "incident-to." Incident-to billing authority allows advanced practice nurses to remain an employee of a physician for "incident-to" services equaling100% of the physician fee schedule (Minarik, 1998).

During the rule-writing process for the above legislation, the definition of "collaboration" was debated. The primary issue surrounding collaboration was the impact of collaboration provisions on practice in states where collaboration is not required and advanced practice nurses can practice independently. The final rules state that in the absence of state law or guidelines governing collaborative relationships, NP must document their scope of practice and "indicate the relationship they have with physicians to deal with issues outside their scope of practice" (Fox, 1998, p. 1). However, how and where this documentation is to be kept is not specified.

An educational requirement for advanced practice nurses was also written into HCFA's final rules. To receive reimbursement a NP must:

- possess a master's degree;
- be a registered professional nurse who is authorized by the state in which the services are furnished to practice as a nurse practitioner in accordance with state law; and
- be certified as a NP by the ANCC or other recognized national certifying bodies that have established standards for NPs (Fox, 1998, p. 2)

These education requirements are a concern for nurse practitioners. The American College of Nurse Practitioners has voiced its concern about the lack of a "grandfathering" clause for certified NPs without a master's degree prior to enactment of the ruling on January 1, 1999. The intent of the law was to provide greater access to NPs for consumers. The master's degree requirement without a grandfathering clause greatly restricts the intent of the original legislation (ACNP, 1998c; Fox, 1998). Resolution of this concern is pending.

In general, PL 105-33 lifted one of the barriers to advanced nursing practice. The legislation is a victory for advanced practice nurses. An NP can obtain information to become a medical provider from the toll-free Social Security telephone number (1-800-772-1213).

Medicaid

Medicaid is a federally supported, state-administered program for low-income families and individuals. Certain groups, such as Aid to Families with Dependent Children (AFDC), low-income elderly, or the disabled are covered under this program. Medicaid is different from Medicare in that it is a vendor program; that is, providers offering services to these individuals or families must accept the Medicaid reimbursement as full payment. Medicaid benefits vary between 70%–100% from state to state. Some states have applied for "Medicaid waivers" allowing states to enroll all Medicaid patients in a MCO (Buppert, 1998).

Section 6405 of OBRA 1989 (PL 101-239) provides for availability and accessibility of services provided by certified pediatric nurse practitioners and certified family nurse practitioners to patients receiving Medicaid. Certification requirements necessary for reimbursement include possession of a current RN license in the state where services are provided; ability to meet state certification requirements; and certification by ANCC as a pediatric nurse practitioner or family nurse practitioner. Pediatric nurse practitioners also may qualify if they are certified by the National Board of Pediatric Nurse Practitioners and Associates.

Indemnity insurers

Health care providers are paid on a per-person, per-procedure basis (Buppert, 1998). Reimbursement is based on "usual and customary charges," which vary from region to region. If the provider charges more than what the insurer allows, the patient is responsible for the difference.

Managed Care Organizations (MCO)

Managed care organizations are growing in the United States. MCOs solicit clients, such as employers, individuals, or governmental agencies, to sell health service packages. Each MCO has a panel of health care providers who may or may not be employed by the MCO (Buppert, 1998). More NPs are applying to become primary care providers (PCP) on MCO provider panels. MCOs reimburse PCPs on a fee-for-service basis, a capitated or fee-per-member basis, or a combination of fee-for-service and capitation. Not all MCOs recognize NPs as PCPs.

One example of the utilization of nurse practitioners as PCPs is the Columbia Advanced Practice Nurse Associates (CAPNA), an independent NP primary care clinic located in a Manhattan neighborhood. CAPNA is listed on the provider panel of several MCOs, and reimbursement is at physician rates. CAPNA is unique in that it is run entirely by NPs.

Other Issues Related to Reimbursement

APNs need to become more knowledgeable in their billing and use of diagnoses. Each patient visit is coded based on Evaluation and Management Service Codes or CPT codes (American Medical Association, 1999). CPT codes is a uniform coding system developed by the American Medical Association and adopted by insurance companies for use in claim submission. CPT codes are based on problem or expanded focus history and examination, complexity of decision making, counseling and minutes of face-to-face-time. CPT codes are associated medical diagnoses based on the International Classification of Diseases (ICD) (American Medical Association, 1998). ICD classification is classified by disease based on medical diagnoses and coded into 6-digit numbers. APNs need to be familiar with ICD codes and correlate documentation with appropriate CPT and ICD codes (Buppert, 1998).

CLINICAL PRIVILEGES

Clinical privileges are defined as "the autonomy to perform expanded role functions based on the individual's licensure, educational preparation, clinical experience and credentials" (Quigley, Hixon, & Janzen, 1991, p. 27). Clinical privileges have been successfully obtained for certified nurse-midwives (CNM) and certified registered nurse anesthe-tists (CRNA). However, clinical privileges in acute care settings for other advanced practice nurses have not been readily obtained. Few institutions provide clinical privileges for advanced practice nurses (Moss, 1993). However, given Medicare reimbursement for NPs in all settings, requests for clinical privileges may significantly improve.

Because of the great diversity in qualifications for APNs, including CRNA and CNMs, it is difficult for agencies to develop clinical privileg-ing guidelines. One area of concern lies in the lack of uniformity in the titles used for APNs. Not only do various terms denote a nurse in ad-vanced practice (i.e., nurse clinician, acute care practitioner, CNS, NP), but variability exists among institutions as to how privileging is used and defined (Hesterly, 1991; Quigley et al., 1991; Smith, 1991; Wehr-hagen & McKiernan, 1991).

The lack of uniformity in medical staff bylaws can create problems for APNs seeking clinical privileges at more than one hospital (Moss, 1993). It is helpful for the APN to request assistance form the Board of Nursing or State Nurses Association to facilitate education of the medical and hospital staff relating to advanced nursing practice related to APN regulation.

Smith (1991) identified four issues encountered in obtaining clinical privileges for APNs. These are:

1) acceptance of the APN by medical and nursing staffs;
2) clear definition and approval of the scope of practice for APN;
3) development of the entry and credentialing process; and
4) revision of hospital and nursing policies to reflect expanded nurs-ing roles (p. 41).

Some physicians and nurses may be resistant to accepting APNs based on the belief that advanced nursing practice oversteps the boundaries of nursing and medicine. Until states provide adequate legislation to define the scope of advanced nursing practice, it will be difficult for institutions to design clin-ical privileging guidelines. The nursing profession must also move quickly to establish a standardized credentialing process and mutually agreed-upon terms to designate APNs. Until these questions are resolved, it will be difficult to change hospital policies to allow APN clinical privileges.

The clinical privileging process used by one institution in New York may be helpful to APNs. The process was facilitated by the New York state legislation which certifies nurse practitioners. Certification by the state of New York includes the granting of prescriptive authority to APNs. Practice agreements and protocols with the collaborating physi-cian, along with a written scope of practice, are also required to obtain advanced practice privileges in this institution. The practice agreements include provisions for resolutions of disagreements between the collaborating physician and nurse practitioners. Verification of liability insurance is also required if the APN is not an employee of the institution. It is noted that this particular institution has different sets of privileges for CNSs and NPs. Patient orders written by CNSs must be countersigned by the physician, whereas this is not a requirement for NPs. Initial privileges are granted for 1 year and are renewed biennially.

Peer review is an important component of the privileging process (Moss, 1993; Smith, 1991). APNs must be active participants in maintaining standards of practice within agencies or institutions. Establishment of a peer-review system may facilitate obtaining clinical privileges for APNs (Moss, 1993).

As advanced practice nurses continue to expand their scope of practice within acute care facilities, clinical privileges will become more important. The process for obtaining clinical privileges will be facilitated by the use of a common language about advanced practice and state legislation regarding scope of practice, particularly prescriptive authority. The placement of nurses in high administrative posts in agencies will facilitate obtaining clinical privileges for nurses. Educating staff, physicians, institutions, and communities regarding advanced nursing practice is necessary before clinical privileges are granted without question for APNs.

LEGISLATIVE INVOLVEMENT

Professional nurses are taking a more active role in the political arena and resulting legislation. Whereas nurses in the past have not been considered a strong voting force, politicians now actively seek the support of local, state, and national nursing organizations. Until recently, most legislators did not recognize the difference between entry-level professional nurses and nurses in advanced practice. This may be due to the fact that nurses in advanced clinical practice, particularly ANPs working in acute care settings, tend to be silent on legislative issues affecting their practice (Mercer, 1993). However, as nurses in advanced practice become highly marketable, issues related to advanced practice will be addressed or reviewed by state legislators. It is essential that nurses in advanced practice communicate with legislators regarding prescriptive authority, second licensure, reimbursement, and legal authority. Although research has demonstrated the cost-effectiveness of advanced practice nurses, state legislation often restricts the ability of APNs to practice autonomously (Smrcina, 1992).

Professional nursing organizations, such as the American Nurses Association (ANA) and American College of Nurse Practitioners (ACNP), facilitate an awareness of legislative issues that directly affect practice. The ANA uses a federation organizational model that requires members join a state nursing association and by virtue of the membership become members of the American Nurses Association. The model provides dual legislative impact. Dual membership supports lobbying efforts both at the state and federal level.

One of the reasons for organizing a strong united effort among advanced practice nurses is the limited financial resources of professional nursing organizations. Professional nursing organizations have approximately $300,000 for lobbying efforts, compared to $3 million offered by medical groups (Inglis & Kjervik, 1993). Since it is difficult to compete financially, the ANA established, Nurses Strategic Action Team (N-STAT) in 1993 to demonstrate unity within the profession. This approach establishes a grass-roots network to provide nurses with greater political clout through strength in numbers. Through this mechanism, it is hoped that nursing's voice will be heard and be rendered as effective as lobbying efforts of other health professions. This grassroots effort was critical to the success of the Medicare reimbursement process.

Legislation can also be influenced by individuals. Writing to state and national legislators is essential to familiarize lawmakers with issues related to advanced practice. Individual efforts, organizational networks, and professional lobbyists advocating support for advanced practice issues provide a strong, united voice for successful passage of advanced practice legislation. Birkholz and Walker (1994) provided helpful suggestions for facilitating legislative action related to advanced practice.

CONCLUSION

Several issues affecting advanced nursing practice have been discussed. All—licensure, certification, prescriptive authority, reimbursement, and clinical privileges—are interrelated. APNs can shape their future by actively participating in the process to resolve these problems. Careful vigilance to legislative action at the state and federal level has resulted in passage of enabling legislation or repealing an unfavorable legislation. APNs must continue to be proactive in efforts to educate legislators, agency administrators, nursing staffs, and the community regarding the scope of advanced practice so that cooperative resolution of issues can occur.

REFERENCES

American Academy of Nurse Practitioners. (1998). *Certification program.* Austin, TX: Author.

American College of Nurse Practitioners. (1998a). Medicare and Medicaid reimbursement for NPs [On-line]. Available: http://www.nurse.org/acnp/facts/reimb.shtml.

American College of Nurse Practitioners. (1998b). Multistate licensure: An update. *ACNP Forum, 1(3),* 7.

American College of Nurse Practitioners. (1998c). Summary of HCFA program memorandum [On-line]. Available: http://www.nurse.org/acnp/medicare/hcfa9804.shtml.

American Medical Association (1998). *International classification of disease.* Dover, DE: Author.

American Medical Association. (1998). *Current procedural terminology.* Chicago, IL: Author.

American Nurses Association. (1993). *The reimbursement manual: How to get paid for your advanced practice nursing services.* Washington, DC: Author.

American Nurses Credentialing Center. (1997a). *Advanced practice certification catalog.* Washington, DC: Author.

American Nurses Credentialing Center. (1997). *Credentialing news.* Washington, DC: Author.

American Nurses Credentialing Center. (1998). *Advanced practice board certification catalog.* Washington, DC: Author.

Birkholz, G., & Walker, D. (1994). Strategies for state statutory language changes granting fully independent nurse practitioner practice. *Nurse Practitioner,* 19, 54–58.

Buppert, C. (1998). Reimbursement for nurse practitioner services. *Nurse Practitioner, 23(1),* 67, 70, 72–76.

Carson, W. (1993). Gains and challenges in prescriptive authority. *American Nurse, 25,* 19–20.

Cassetta, R. A. (1993). Opening doors for advanced practice opportunities. *American Nurse, 25,* 18–19.

Federal Register. (1992). Definition and registration of mid-level practitioners: 21 CFR Parts 1301 and 1304. *Federal Register, 57*(146), 33465.

Ferguson, S. (1996). The use of Medicaid managed care: A case study of two states. *Journal of Pediatric Nursing, 11,* 189–191.

Finefrock, W., & Hardy Havens, D. (1997). Coverage and reimbursement issues for nurse practitioners. *Journal of Pediatric Health Care, 11,* 139–142.

Fox, A. (1998). Analysis report: HCFA Final Rule. *American College of Nurse Practitioners.* Report #202-546-4825.

Hesterly, S. C. (1991). Nurse credentialing in an acute care setting. *Journal of Nursing Quality Assurance, 5*(3), 18–26.

Inglis, A. D., & Kjervik, D. K. (1993). Empowerment of advanced practice nurses: Regulation reform needed to increase access to care. *The Journal of Law, Medicine & Ethics, 21,* 193–205.

Malone, B. (1993). Second licensure? ANA and NCSBN debate the issue. *The American Nurse, 25,* 8.

Mercer, M. (1993, May). *Advanced practice: Looking to the year 2000.* Paper presented at the American Association of Critical Care Nurses National Teaching Institute, Anaheim, CA.

Minarik, P.A. (1998). Medicare and Medicaid reimbursement: New law and new legislation. *Clinical Nurse Specialist, 12*(2), 83–84.

Mittelstadt, P. (1998). Federal reimbursement of advanced practice nurses' services empowers the profession. *Nurse Practitioner, 18*(1), 43–49.

Mirr, M. P. (1981). *The evolution of the Wisconsin nurse practice act.* Unpublished master's thesis, University of Wisconsin-Madison.

Moss, R. W. (1993). Privileging essential to APN autonomy. *The American Nurse, 25,* 7, 21.

Omnibus Budget Reconciliation Act 1989. (December 19). P.L. 101–239, H. R. 3299, Section 6213.

Pearson, L. J. (1999). Annual update of how each state stands on legislative issues affecting advanced nursing practice. *Nurse Practitioner, 24*(1), 14–66.

Quigley, P., Hixon, A. K., & Janzen, S. K. (1991). Promoting autonomy and professional practice: A program of clinical privileging. *Journal of Nursing Quality Assurance, 5*(3), 27–32.

Sheets, V. R. (1993). Second licensure? ANA and NCSBN debate the issue. *The American Nurse, 25,* 8–9.

Smith, T. C. (1991). A structural process to credential nurses with advanced practice skills. *Journal of Nursing Quality Assurance, 5,* 40–51.

Smrcina, C. (1992). Public policy issues: Advanced practice and health care reform: What should you do? *Orthopaedic Nursing, 11,* 7.

Wehrhagen, R., & McKiernan, N. A. (1991). Credentialing and clinical privileging: Experiences at a tertiary care center. *Journal of Nursing Quality Assurance, 5,* 33–39.

Chapter 4

SETTINGS FOR PRACTICE: WORKING WITHIN A CHANGING HEALTH CARE SYSTEM

Mary Zwygart-Stauffacher, PhD, RN, CS, GNP/GCNS
Linda Lindeke, PhD, RN, CPNP

INTRODUCTION

The health care system has undergone tremendous change during recent decades: the emergence of Diagnostic Related Groups (DRGs), prospective payment systems, decreased hospital stays, and managed care, coupled with the explosion of home health care programs and alternative health care. The result is the development of a new and rapidly changing health care system, ripe for molding by the advanced practice nurse, yet, also possibly a daunting undertaking to many. The Advanced Practice Nurse (APN) who was traditionally educated to provide advanced nursing more closely aligned to a specific system or setting of care, now is faced with the challenge of a multisystem arena for care delivery. Not only are the settings of care rapidly changing, but the methods for reimbursement are also complex and evolving. The advantages and challenges of traditional third-party payers' fees for service are now joined with the need for understanding and negotiating the managed care environment and the capitated health care delivery systems. Nurses who frequently were familiar with the nonprofit orientation of health care are now faced with the need to understand the economics of health care and the health care systems. Therefore, understanding system issues has been identified as necessary not only in education of nurse administrators, but also for the APN. As a component of a study by Lynn, Layman, and Englebardt (1998), the importance of advanced practice education programs incorporating nursing administration content was identified. This includes content in areas such as leadership, financial management, politics, and health policy. The delivery of care by the APN has also included concern for and commitment to the uninsured and underinsured. Within the competitive health care arena, the needs of these consumers must not be forgotten. Nurses have been pivotal in the establishment of community clinics and free clinics, yet they will be challenged to achieve that social justice commitment in the future.

CHANGING AND CHALLENGING ISSUES AND TRENDS

The Changing Health Care System

Over the past decade, numerous changes have occurred in the delivery of health care services. In an attempt to achieve cost savings, mergers of health care organizations have given birth to giant health care corporations. However, the demonstrated cost savings have not necessarily been consistently and nationally achieved. Other initiatives have also been instituted to achieve health care cost savings, such as shorter lengths of stays in hospitals, increased patient visits in outpatient clinics, and increased use of subacute facilities. These "quick fix" ideas have often created new and challenging problems. For example, most subacute facilities were not designed or staffed for the level of acuity that "subacute" has come to mean.

Despite an increased emphasis on wellness and prevention, managed care has resulted in decreased primary care health screening and fewer routine physical examinations. Rarely is the emphasis in managed care systems placed on receiving care from a consistent provider in both health and illness. Urgent care clinics have removed the continuity of care component from ambulatory care. This lack of continuity in care is also affected by employers constantly changing health plans in order to renegotiate better benefit contracts. When employees frequently have to change provider systems due to contract changes, they do not establish trusting relationships with providers or become familiar with systems to know where to go for care. The emphasis on the importance of primary care, articulated in the early 1990s by groups such as the Institute of Medicine, has certainly been diminished by, if not lost, due to many economic factors.

Nursing Trends

Coupled with the changes in the delivery system is the shift in the nursing work force. The Division of Nursing (1996) reports that the nursing work force is aging. In 1996, only 9% of the 2.5 million United States (U.S.) registered nurse (RN) workforce was below the age of 30, with the average age of RNs being 44 years of age. This is in comparison to 1980 data, at which time the average age was 40. At a time when systems need highly educated nurses with bachelors and master's preparation, 60% of U.S. nursing graduates graduated from associate degree nursing programs. The workforce issue is compounded when considering the conclusions reported in a recent AACN report in which specialty practice nurses are most needed in this country, specifically nurses in psychiatry, pediatric cancer care, and community health (AACN, 1998). Gerontologic nurse practitioners, neonatal nurse practitioners, and those with cardiovascular and neurologic nursing skills are also in short supply.

Managed Care

Managed care has developed rapidly in the 1990s in response to many economic and political forces. There is a paradigm shift in health care delivery occurring, and this will continue regardless of whether health care reform legislation is passed in the future (Issel & Anderson, 1996). Congress did not pass the 1993 Clinton health care reform initiative.

This failure led to rapid mergers of health systems, formation of integrated service delivery networks, and competitive contracting by employers with service providers—all in the effort to develop systems to decrease rapidly escalating health care costs. As a result, American health care has adopted the "bottom-line," profit/loss mentality of the business world.

Demographics indicate that the U.S. post-World War II "baby-boom" generation is transitioning into middle age. This large increase in the percentage of the population which is growing older and of high consumers of health care is a trend that is projected to continue into the 21st century. The enormous costs of emerging technologies used in providing care to elders are bankrupting Medicare funds. This has resulted in even greater use of managed care strategies for Medicare recipients in an attempt to control health care costs. The U.S. health care system has many dissatisfied care providers and worried patients within managed care organizations. These latter organizations are huge, complex, and have been unable to demonstrate the expected cost savings. Some managed care strategies, such as employing economies of scale in purchasing, centralizing services such as emergency care, and developing systems for referrals and after-hours care have been cost-effective. However politicians are skeptical about the quality of care provided. The general public is confused, as they have had to negotiate with constantly changing health care systems in order to obtain decreasing numbers of health care services. "Managed care" is frequently interpreted as "managed costs." Increased regulation by the Health Care Financing Agency (HCFA) in an effort to uncover Medicare/Medicaid fraud has added to the negative light in which providers and consumers view recent health care system changes. APNs are also voicing their discomfort with the changes, particularly about the expectations of some managed care organizations to limit the length of patient visits to 10 to 15 minutes. In high-production models of care, APNs may not be able to fulfill their responsibility to prevent illness and to teach patients about their treatment plans.

Interdisciplinary Teams

Teams have received a great deal of emphasis in workplace redesign, partially because of the successes of teams in the corporate world. The costs of teams must be factored into health care delivery models. Each team member must contribute fully in order for the expense of the collaboration of multiple providers to be justified. Therefore, advanced practice nurses must function from a clear understanding of the nursing discipline in order for their contribution to be unique and cost-effective.

Three qualities are essential to the effective functioning of health care teams.

1. Each member has a unique contribution to make to the team,
2. Each member is competent in a particular role,
3. Members understand what each person contributes and honor the contribution of each member.

McCloskey and Maas (1998) caution teams against adopting "group think," where the members are focused more on relationships and getting along than on the need to clearly articulate their individual perspectives. They also urge nurses not to be so focused on interdisciplinary methods and processes that the unique role of nursing is blurred or irretrievable from the group outcome data.

Collaboration is the term of choice for advanced practice nurses working in interdisciplinary teams, as it avoids any sense of one health care discipline supervising the work of another. Collaboration suggests discipline-specific knowledge and responsibilities of each team member, acknowledging that there are areas in which the disciplines overlap or that provider skills may be interchangeable. Nurse practice acts have typically contained language allowing registered nurses to carry out delegated medical functions. This has allowed nurses to expand their scope of practice into new areas. However, it is essential that APN knowledge, skills, and practice not be seen as "delegated medical functions." The evolvement of the advanced practice nursing role has been partially a process of demonstrating to the nursing profession, other professionals, and the public that APNs function autonomously based on a discipline-specific knowledge base. It is therefore not appropriate to bring supervisory relationships into the process of patient care delivered by teams.

The language of collaboration is vital to the success of teams as well as to the description and evaluation of health care outcomes. McCloskey and Maas (1998) have very specific concerns regarding the value of discipline-specific language (such as embodied in NANDA, NIC, and NOC) being overlooked in the rush to develop a single language shared by all health care disciplines. In this era of computerized record-keeping systems for health care, physicians have used systems such as Current Procedure Terminology (CPT) and International Classification of Diseases-9th Edition (ICD-9) which describe characteristics of their practice. However, these medical coding systems do not focus on outcomes of care or specific interventions. APNs on interdisciplinary teams face the challenge of bringing the focus constantly back to a holistic view of the patient and to articulate and demonstrate specific nursing outcomes within the collaborative effort.

Effect of Reimbursement on Health Delivery Systems

The changing health care delivery system is dramatically altering the types of organizations where nurses work and thus the methods by which nurses are reimbursed. Factors motivating this change are financial forces and concerns about the continuing rise in the cost of health care. Therefore it is pivotal that advanced practice nurses have knowledge about reimbursement issues and be able to provide leadership in establishing the regulations for reimbursement. The reader is referred to Chapter 3 for further discussion on reimbursement issues. APNs are more likely than staff nurses to individually negotiate their employment contracts, an aspect which affects reimbursement. Additionally, tracking APN cost-effectiveness, productivity, and fiscal outcomes of nursing care is essential to the entire nursing profession as well as to its individual practitioners. Measuring outcomes is one of the highest health care priorities of the current era. APNs must be informed about and active in outcome research and practice endeavors (Buerhaus, 1998; Buppert, 1998).

Many forces impact APN reimbursement (see Figure 4.1), making reimbursement a complex issue. The fiscal structure of health care is rapidly changing, requiring APNs to continually update their knowledge of these issues. Multiple forces, which are often political in nature, are played out in Congress as well as in each state legislature, within county governments, and at the APN worksite in employment agreements and organizational policies. Examining the various forces individually assists APNs in directing attention to the appropriate entity.

The American public has three overriding concerns regarding health care: access, cost, and quality. The United States is unique in having a health care system where provider competition is a driving force. Additionally, 50 different state-specific configurations of health care exist as most reimbursement laws and policies are developed at the state level. Currently over, 43 million individuals in the United States lack health care coverage (New York Times, Sept. 26, 1998). Some of those individuals choose to self-insure, some are unable or unwilling to negotiate the bureaucracy necessary to obtain coverage from public programs for which

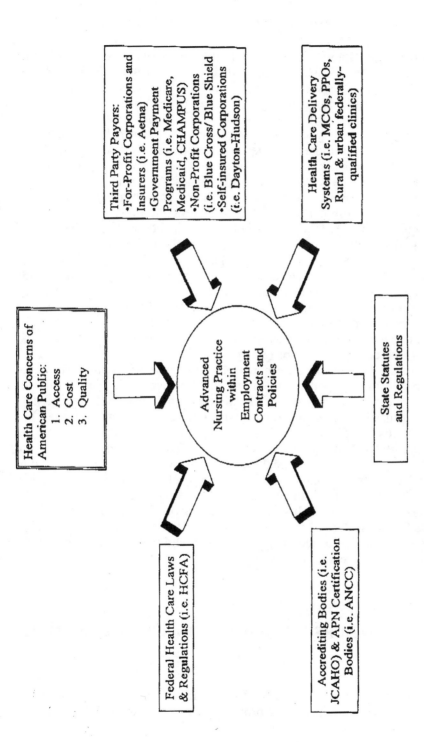

FIGURE 4.1 Reimbursement Realities for Advanced Practice Nurses

they are eligible, and others are ineligible for public or employer-based coverage, frequently because of part-time employment. Access to care for the uninsured, as well as the underinsured, remains a pressing issue. Even Americans with insurance have concerns about access to care. Many health plans restrict access to specialty care by having primary care providers act as gatekeepers through a system of referrals and prior authorization for the more costly health care components. Additionally, health plans limit the providers to their salaried staff in staff-model HMOs, or to a contracted list of specialists and agencies. Thus, Americans with and without health care coverage have concerns about access to needed care.

Quality of health care in the US is also a continuing public concern. This concern has recently been expressed in federal legislative efforts for a Patient Bill of Rights, thus articulating the rights of patients to sue and obtain care in Managed Care Organizations (MCOs). A highly debated issue in the proposed legislation is the patient's right to sue MCOs for denied or inadequate care. This legislative initiative is based on public perception that quality of care has declined in the MCO quest for a balanced bottom line. Cuts in Medicare and Medicaid spending have also increased public concern that quality of care may be affected and access reduced in the future (Sharp, 1997).

Cost of care continues to increase, making the American health care system the most expensive in the world. Managed care temporarily reduced the rate of increase of health care cost. However, recent data indicate that increased demand for specialty care and the increased use of high-cost medical technology are increasing costs and decreasing profitability of managed care corporations. The US spends 14% of the Gross National Product on health care, with an upward trend expected to continue as the population ages. The cost-effectiveness of APNs has been well documented, therefore APNs are in demand in managed care organizations (Cohen & Juszczak, 1997; Mason, Cohen, O'Connel, Baxter, & Chase, 1997; Schaffner & Bohomey, 1998). Systems can be put in place to assist NPs to measure productivity and thereby track cost-effectiveness of their care (Kearns, 1992).

ADVANCED NURSING PRACTICE IN SPECIFIC SETTINGS

Current emphasis on continuity of care will increasingly result in APNs moving across settings as they provide care. For example, NPs may have hospital privileges and continue to care for their ambulatory patients during periods of hospitalization. Similarly, CNSs may at times care for their clients as they progress through inpatient, outpatient, and long-term care settings. Collaboration among APNs in various settings is critical to the continuity of care. Therefore, it is important for APNs to have an understanding about traditional and emerging roles and functions of APNs in many settings. Many new opportunities for APNs are emerging.

Acute Care

High patient acuity with shorter hospital stays, along with downsized hospital staffs and high technological skill requirements, has led the way for expanded advanced practice roles in the acute care setting. The decrease in the number of resident physician positions available in specialty practices has contributed to new opportunities for APNs (Clochesy, Daly, Idemoto, Steel, & Fitzpatrick, 1994; Dracup & Bryan-Brown, 1994; Keane, Richmond, & Kaiser, 1994). APNs provide consistency and a holistic patient perspective that rotating medical house staff often cannot provide.

The clinical nurse specialist role (CNS) was developed in the 1960s. As reported by Christman (1991), these nursing specialists provide a high level of specialized care and serve as change agents in hospital settings through role modeling and consultation with other providers. Whereas CNSs have contributed to the quality of patient care in acute care settings for the past three decades, changes in the delivery of care are creating new avenues for APNs. For instance, APNs working as discharge planners have been shown to reduce costs and improve care outcomes (Naylor, 1990; Vaska, 1993). Increased patient acuity in hospitals requires that APNs possess advanced technical skills as well as expertise in physiological and psychosocial realms. APNs can assist staff in making clinical decisions about treatment options for acutely ill patients (Gleeson et al., 1990); Sawyers, 1993; Schroer, 1991).

An example of a new role is the development of the Acute Care Nurse Practitioner (ACNP). This role is not to be a replacement for CNSs, but a new role for advanced practice nurses within acute care settings. The primary focus of this new APN role in inpatient settings is to provide comprehensive, direct patient care from admission to discharge (Gleeson et al., 1990; Haddad, 1992; Hunsberger et al., 1992; Niemela, Poster,

& Moreau, 1992). APN activities include comprehensive admission assessment with history-taking and physical examination, coordination and implementation of care by ordering and interpreting diagnostics, and implementing and evaluating interventions. Emphasis on continuity of care as patients move across settings requires that acute care nurse practitioners be skilled in the coordination of care.

Demand for ACNPs is being created by a shortage of physician residents in hospitals, as result of the Physicians Payment Review Commission (PPRC) recommendation to limit specialty residency positions (Keane et al., 1994). ACNP roles occur primarily in inpatient settings such as neonatal intensive care, critical care, psychiatry, pediatrics, and adult specialty units. Many neonatal intensive care units have employed nurse practitioners for several years, and have had positive patient outcomes and cost-saving from these collaborative efforts (Bissinger, Allred, Arford, & Bellig, 1997; Dracup & Bryan-Brown, 1994).

Acute care practitioners have been placed within organizations mainly in two ways: 1) Employment in a unit- or service-based program, such as a liver transplant unit, or 2) employment in a professional practice model, where APNs joins physician practices or groups and assume care responsibilities within those practice (Keane et al., 1994). Vaska (1993) describes her role as an ACNP in cardiovascular surgery as being the case manager for cardiac surgery patients. In collaboration with surgeons, she assesses, plans, and implements preoperative and postoperative care. She makes daily rounds on patients and follows their progress using an integrated clinical pathway as a tool for standardized care. One of the more positive results from this position has been the early discharge planning initiated by the APN. Since the position was implemented, the length of stay for the average cardiac surgery patient was decreased by 2.02 days with a decrease in total cost of $1,445.34 (Vaska, 1993, p. 643). The success of the collaborative practice model with physicians and nurse practitioners in the acute care setting was more recently demonstrated by the practice model implemented at the University of Missouri Health Sciences Center (Knaus, Felten, Burton, Fobes, & Davis, 1997). They documented the appropriateness of use of NPs in acute care settings.

Early discharge planning by APNs, some of whom are also designated as discharge planning nurses, has been shown to be effective in reducing health care costs as well as resulting in positive patient outcomes. Research by Brooten et al. (1986) on early discharge of low birth weight infants that was coordinated and planned by APNs demonstrated significant cost savings. Naylor's (1990) work with comprehensive discharge planning for the hospitalized elderly has also demonstrated positive patient outcomes and cost savings.

Acute care nurse practitioners in critical care specialties are currently the fastest-growing APN specialty. Many academic institutions are responding to the need for ACPNs (Clochesy et al., 1994) and are initiating graduate nursing programs of study. ACNPs in critical care provide direct patient care management, including admission and discharge, history and physicals, evaluating clinical data, planning and prescribing treatment plans, using invasive procedures when needed, working with families, and coordinating care (Keane et al., 1994). Certification is available within a national credentialing center (American Nurses Credentialing Center) for acute care practitioners in adult health. Work has also begun to develop an ACNP in pediatrics. It is important to note that the first such acute care practitioner examination was the certification of the neonatal nurse practitioner by the National Certification Corporation (NCC) for the Obstetrics, Gynecologic and Neonatal Nursing Specialties.

APNs will continue to function in acute care settings in the more traditional CNS role as well as the newly developing and expanding role, the ACNP. With changes in health care delivery and reimbursement, there has been speculation that traditional CNS positions would be eliminated or modified to incorporate a broader and more direct patient care role. Though this has been operationalized in some settings, this has not occurred nationally at the rate expected by some nursing leaders. In fact, there has been a recent resurgence of discussion as to whether it is appropriate and reasonable to attempt to educate nurses who can merge the CNS and NP roles within a 2-year graduate nursing program.

Long-term care

The elderly, those 65 years of age and older, are the fastest growing segment of the population. The sheer numbers of elderly, coupled with the likelihood of the development of chronic illness as persons age, present a challenge to society. The care issues of this population require tremendous resources. Although much of the care of this population occurs outside of nursing homes, care of residents in nursing homes exceeds $35 billion health care dollars a year (Maddox, 1994). APNs possess the knowledge and skills to provide quality health care for elders, particularly those in long-term care facilities or nursing homes.

McDougall and Roberts (1993) suggested that an APN in every nursing home is a necessary expenditure. Studies have shown that the use of NPs in nursing homes has resulted in earlier detection of problems, increased resident satisfaction (Kane et al., 1988), decreased hospitalizations of residents (Garrard et al., 1990), and reduced prescriptions for medications (Patrick, Davignon, Enloe, & Milburn, 1990). According to Mezey and Lynaugh (1991), having an NP in every nursing home would result in cost savings of over a billion dollars a year. However, nursing homes have struggled with the cost of adding APNs to the staffing ratio. This is due to the lack of ability for nursing homes to bill for APN services if the APNs are employed by the facility. If employed by nursing homes, regulatory statutes view APNs as members of the nursing staff; APN services are therefore considered to be a dimension of the nursing home reimbursement payment. If APNs were to generate separate billings, it would be viewed as double-billing for their service.

APNs in long-term care facilities have implemented their practice in a variety of modes. Facility-based APNs, who at times provide primary care for residents, frequently function in the roles of consultants and facilitators in planning nursing care for residents, educating staff, and evaluating the quality of care provided. Teaching long-term care staff, particularly the nonprofessional staff, is a key role of APNs in nursing homes. Because few professional nurses are present in nursing homes, role modeling by APNs provides nursing staff, both professional and nonprofessional, with direction of care delivery and care evaluation.

A number of innovative systems have evolved for the delivery of nurse practitioner services in long-term care. One of these is Evercare, which is based in Minneapolis, MN. Within this program, Evercare provides primary care for frail elderly nursing home residents. Each NP, with a collaborating physician, has a caseload of approximately 110 residents. Rounds are made on a routine basis, with nursing home staff utilizing the NP as the first-line contact about problems and changes in a resident's condition. Evercare and similar nursing home services programs have demonstrated that the GNP can handle the vast majority of problems/concerns that arise in nursing homes.

Medicare regulations prohibiting reimbursement for APNs who provide primary care for nursing home residents had previously been a barrier to greater use of NPs in long-term care facilities (McDougall & Roberts, 1993; Nichols, 1992). However, with federal legislative changes, this has become much less of an issue. Reimbursement for APN visits to longterm care is set at 85% of the typical fee for physicians. This reimbursement is only for certified APNs who work in collaboration with a physician or physician groups. With this collaborative team approach, the team is able to bill for nursing home services more frequently than can a physician-only practice.

Though the vast majority of elderly residents residing in nursing homes will live out the remainder of their lives at the home, there is an increasing number of short-term stay nursing home residents, such as patients requiring palliative care or rehabilitation. This is another role arena for APNs, and an area in which APNs can be more greatly utilized. Demonstration of the usefulness of the APN to enhance quality care in a cost effective basis is required in the subacute care settings.

Home and Community Settings Care

To date, APNs have not been employed extensively in home care, hospice care, or other community-related health services. Barriers to practice in nontraditional settings, such as reimbursement and various prescriptive privileges, are gradually being removed. However, many opportunities exist for APNs to contribute significantly to the care of persons receiving health care in their homes (Beuscher, 1994). Early hospital discharges requires that home care nurses be highly knowledgeable about technology as well as being superb educators and decision makers. Greater attention is being given to the types of assistance that persons with chronic illnesses, particularly older persons, need to remain in their own homes or in senior housing or assisted living facilities, rather than in nursing homes. Home visits by APNs facilitate access to care when clients are unable to travel to clinics. Because many of these persons have chronic conditions warranting continued monitoring of treatment, home visits by APNs may decrease costs. Lack of reimbursement for these home visits, which can serve as replacements for ambulatory visits, has limited the utilization of primary care APN services in the home.

Beuscher (1994) provides a compelling description of her role as an APN for two rural community-based residential facilities (CBRF). She relates how she visits each facility weekly and conducts monthly assessments of each resident. Minor treatments and preventive care have resulted in cost savings and convenience for the facilities and residents.

APNs may serve as case managers for caseloads of clients in home care settings. One setting in which this has occurred is the Veteran's Administration home-based health care service. Activities of APNs include conducting comprehensive assessment with an initial history-taking and physical examination, prescribing the treatment regimen, monitoring and interpreting diagnostic tests, ordering immunizations, and making referrals. Care is coordinated with other health care providers and is based on both nursing and medical diagnoses (Schroer, 1991).

For over three decades psychiatric-mental health APNs have been key members of mental health teams providing care in communities. Psychiatric-mental health APNs are prepared to provide therapy to individuals and families, serve as group leaders of family therapy or support groups, and provide consultation to other health care providers about mental health problems. APNs who are prepared in psychiatric-mental health nursing are sorely needed to address the needs of the growing number of persons with chronic mental health problems, alcohol and drug abuse, physical and sexual abuse, and dementia.

Another example of APNs addressing special needs populations is in the care of medically fragile adolescents (Dougherty, 1992). The APN works with schools to assess the educational, psychological, and medical needs of a group of adolescents with chronic illnesses. The holistic APN perspective and thorough history-taking physical examination skills uncover many health needs that had previously not been addressed, because attention tends to focus solely on the chief chronic condition.

> a current nursing care delivery model that practices holistic health care. Parish nurses provide care to a faith community, emphasizing the relationship between faith and health. Specific nursing activities addres physical, emotional, and spiritual health and well-being, closely attending to the inseparability of these dimensions. (Berquist & King, 1994)

As churches are becoming more aware of their role in caring for the total person, the number of parish nurses is increasing. Concurrently, colleges of nursing are recognizing this need and developing graduate-level educational programs of study. Parish nurses function independently and address a wide variety of health concerns. Those parish nurses who have been educated as APNs possess the unique knowledge and skills to address the health concerns of parishioners. The growing number of elders is one population who is benefiting from the expertise of an APN prepared parish nurse.

Dying with dignity and in comfort is the goal of palliative and hospice care programs. APNs, with their superb assessment skills and interactional skills, can do much to promote comfort in this population. Not only do APNs coordinate the care of the dying person, but they can assist the family in dealing with the loss and the grieving process.

Ambulatory Care Settings

One of the more common setting in which APNs work is primary care settings, especially working collaboratively with physicians in hospital-based clinics or physician offices. These APNs carry a caseload within their general, specialty, or subspecialty practice, referring patients to collaborating physicians when needed.

Specialty clinics have utilized APNs in various role functions. For example, an oncology APN facilitates the administration and follow up care of chemotherapy. These multidimensional follow-up visits consist of physical assessments, functional assessments, and evaluation of toxicities related to therapy (Sawyers, 1993). The oncology APN, traditionally in the role of the CNS, coordinates patient care and involves the house staff, nursing service, social service, and discharge planners as needed. Because APNs bring a holistic perspective to the care of these clients and their families, both the physiological and psychosocial aspects of care are addressed.

Aiken et al. (1993) demonstrated that nurse practitioner-managed care for persons with HIV infections in a large university hospital outpatient clinic has comparable patient outcomes when compared to physician care. APNs reported more patient symptoms related to HIV infection over a given period than physicians. Patients managed by APNs also reported fewer problems with their care.

The development of urgent care departments has provided an additional setting for APNs. This hybrid role deals with the nonemergent care as well as needs previously addressed in the emergency department and walk-in clinics. Urgent care sites have evolved as care delivery settings, where APNs may carve a new role as they assess and treat the many minor acute illnesses with which patients present. Referrals to primary care providers may result from urgent-care visits when APNs detect other health problems requiring attention. Barger (1993) describes an APN who organized and implemented an ambulatory care center for adults with acute and chronic medical or minor trauma problems in a large urban county hospital. The APN used her advanced practice skills to addresses the consequence of violent and unhealthy behaviors. One strategy employed by the APN was the inclusion of the patient and family in the plan of care.

Increased attention is being given to prevention and health promotion, the cornerstone of primary care for APNs. Many health-promoting activities occur in ambulatory care settings. However, it is difficult to accomplish activities related to prevention and promotion during the short time frames such as those that are currently afforded for physician clinic visits in managed care delivery models. Safriet (1992), for example, described how the health care system has given attention to short-term outcomes. She stated that APNs have encountered problems when they have given extended time to clients who seek information about underlying causes of health problems. Providing education and counseling clients to change behaviors takes time and repeated contacts. Studies have shown, however, that such activities have resulted in positive long-term outcomes that would result in cost savings over time (Safriet, 1992). Therefore, health care system changes are necessary for APNs to be truly effective in ambulatory settings.

CONCLUSION

The content provided in this chapter provides for an overview of the challenges and rewards for APNs in various health care settings. The health care systems of the past will no longer exist, but the lessons learned can give direction for future APN role in the emerging system of care. APNs will need to be able to maneuver within ever-changing care systems to assure access, quality and cost-effectiveness of care for their clients.

REFERENCES

Aiken, L., Lake, E., Semaan, S., Lehman, H., O'Hare, P., Cole, C., Dunbar, D., & Frank, I. (1993). Nurse practitioner managed care for persons with HIV infection. *IMAGE: Journal of Nursing Scholarship, 25,* 172–177.

American Association of Colleges of Nursing. (1998). 1997–1998 enrollment and graduations in baccalaureate and graduate programs in nursing. Washington, DC: Author.

Barger, C. (1993). Mary Hale: Serving her community. *Nurse Practitioner Forum, 4,* 182–183.

Bergquist, S., & King, J. (1994). Parish nursing. *Journal of Holistic Nursing, 12,* 155–170.

Beuscher, T. (1994). CBRF's benefit from nursing knowledge. *Nursing Matters, 5*(4), 8.

Bissinger, R., Allred, C., Arford, P., & Bellig, L. (1997). A cost-effectiveness analysis of neonatal nurse practitioners. *Nursing Economics, 15*(2), 92–99.

Brooten, D., Kumar, S., Brown, L., Butts, P., Finker, S., Bakewell-Sachs, S., & Gibbons, A. (1986). A randomized clinical trial of early hospital discharge and home follow-up of very low birth weight infants. *New England Journal of Medicine, 35,* 934–939.

Buerhaus, P. (1998) Medicare payment for advanced practice nurses: What are the research questions? *Nursing Outlook, 46,* 151–153.

Buerhaus, P., & Staiger, D. (1997). Future of the nurse labor market according to health executives in the high managed-care areas of the United States. *Image, 29,* 313–18.

Buppert, C. (1998). Reimbursement for nurse practitioner services. *Nurse Practitioner, 28*(2), 67, 70, 72–76, 81–2.

Christman, L. (1991). Advance nursing practice: Future of clinical nurse specialists. In L. Aiken & C. Fagin (Eds). *Charting nursing's future: Agenda for the 1990's* (pp. 108–120). New York: Lippincott.

Clochesy, J., Daly, B., Idemoto, B., Steel, J., & Fitzpatrick, J. (1994). Preparing advanced practice nurses for acute care. *American Journal of Critical Care, 3,* 255–259.

Cohen, S. & Juszczak, L. (1997). Promoting the nurse practitioner role in managed care. *Journal of Pediatric Health Care, 11,* 3–11.

Dougherty, J. (1992). Wendy Berry: Pediatric nurse practitioner providing care to adolescents with special needs. *Nurse Practitioner Forum, 3,* 187–88.

Dracup, K., & Bryan-Brown, C. (1994). The advanced practice nurse in critical care: Yes or no? *American Journal of Critical Care, 3,* 163–164.

Garrard, J., Kane, R., Radosevich, D., Skay, C., Arnold, S., Kepferle, L., McDermott, S., & Buchanan, J. (1990). Impact of geriatric nurse practitioners on nursing home resident's functional status, satisfaction, and discharge outcomes. *Medical Care, 28,* 271–283.

Gleeson, M., McIlvain-Simpson, G., Boos, M., Sweet, E., Trzcinski, K., Solberg, C., & Doughty, R. (1990). Advanced practice nursing: A model of collaborative care. *Maternal Child Nursing, 15*(1), 9–12.

Haber, J. (1997). Medicare reimbursement: A victory for APRNs. *AJN, 97*(11), 84.

Haddad, B. (1992). Report on the expanded role nurse project. *Canadian Journal of Nursing Administration, 5*(4), 10–17.

Hunsberger, M., Mitchell, A., Blatz, S., Paes, B., Pinelli, J., Southwell, D., French, S., & Soluk, R., (1992). Definition of an advanced nursing practice role in the NICU: The clinical nurse specialist/neonatal practitioner. *Clinical Nurse Specialist, 6,* 91–96.

Issel, L., & Anderson, R. (1996). Take charge: Managing six transformations in health care delivery. *Nursing Economics, 14*(2), 78–85.

Kane, R., Kane, R., Arnold, S., Garrard, J., McDermott, S., & Kepferle, L. (1988). Geriatric nurse practitioners as nursing home employees: Implementing the role. *Gerontologist, 28,* 469–477.

Keane A., Richmond, T., & Kaiser, L. (1994). Critical care nurse practitioners: Evolution of the advanced practice nursing role. *American Journal of Critical Care, 3,* 232–237.

Kearns, D. (1992). A productivity tool to evaluate NP practice: Monitoring clinical time spent in reimbursable, patient-related activities. *Nurse Practitioner, 17*(4), 50–55.

Knaus, V., Felten, S., Burton, S., Fobes, P., & Davis, K. (1997). The use of nurse practitioners in the acute care setting. *Journal of Nursing Administration, 27*(2), 20–27.

Lynn, M., Layman, E., & Englebardt, S. (1998). Nursing administration research priorities a national delphi study. *Journal of Nursing Administration, 28*(5), 7–11.

Maddox, C. (1994). Sociology of aging. In W. Hazzard, E. Bierman, J. Blass, W. Ettinger, & E. Halter (Eds.). *Principles of geriatric medicine and gerontology* (pp. 125–134). New York: McGraw-Hill.

Mason, D., Cohen, S., O-Donnell, J., Baxter, K., & Chase, A. (1997). Managed care organizations' arrangements with nurse practitioners. *Nursing Economics, 15,* 306–14.

McCloskey, J. C., & Maas, M. (1998). Interdisciplinary team: The nursing perspective is essential. *Nursing Outlook, 46,* 157–163.

McDougall, G., & Roberts, B. (1993). A gerontologic nurse practitioner in every home: A necessary expenditure. *Geriatric Nursing, 14,* 218–220.

Mezey, M., & Lynaugh, J. (1991), Teaching nursing home program: A lesson in quality. *Geriatric Nursing, 12,* 76–77.

Naylor, M. (1990). Comprehensive discharge planning for hospitalized elderly: A pilot study. *Nursing Research, 39,* 156–61.

Pear, R. (1998). Americans lacking health insurance put at *New York Times,* Sept 26, 1998.

Nichols, L. M. (1992). Estimating costs of underusing advanced practice nurses. *Nursing Economics, 10,* 343–351.

Niemela, K., Poster, R., & Moreau, D. (1992). The attending nurse: A new role for the advanced clinician. *The Journal of Child and Adolescent Psychiatric and Mental Health Nursing, 5*(3), 5–12.

Patrick, M., Davignon, D., Enloe, C., & Milburn, P. (1990). Prescription for the high cost of drugs in nursing homes. *Geriatric Nursing, 11,* 88–89.

Safriet, B. (1992). Health care dollars and regulatory sense: The role of advanced practice nursing. *Yale Journal on Regulation, 9,* 419–487.

Sawyers, J. (1993). Defining your role in ambulatory care: Clinical nurse specialist or nurse practitioner? *Clinical Nurse Specialist, 7,* 4–7.

Schaffner, R., & Bohomey, J. (1998). Demonstrating APN value in a capitated market. *Nursing Economics, 16,* 69–74.

Schroer, D. (1991). Case management: Clinical nurse specialist and nurse practitioner, converging roles. *Clinical Nurse Specialist, 5,* 189–194.

Vaska, P. (1993). The clinical nurse specialist in cardiovascular surgery: A new twist. *AACN Clinical Issues in Critical Care Nursing, 4,* 637–644.

Chapter **5**

CLINICAL DECISION MAKING

Sheila Corcoran-Perry, PhD, RN, FAAN
Suzanne Narayan, PhD, RN
Marsha Lewis, PhD, RN*

Janet J. Bender, a gerontological nurse practitioner at Sunny-vale Nursing Home, is working with Sarah Vogel, a new resident who is demanding to return to independent living in her apartment. Other staff members have tried to persuade Sarah that the nursing home is the best place for her, but Sarah "doesn't buy it." Sarah's niece, Mary, her only living relative, admitted her to Sunnyvale after she fell at home and wasn't able to get up. Mary indicated that Sarah seems confused at times and doesn't take her medications as prescribed. Mary fears that Sarah is not safe alone. Both Mary and the staff are exasperated with Sarah's demands to "go home." Janet has several lively interactions with Sarah and comes to appreciate her feistiness and determination. She senses that Sarah might be able to live independently. She feels that Sarah de-

*The authors want to acknowledge the contributions of Helen Moreland, MS, RN, CS and Carol O'Boyle, PhD, RN for their assistance in developing the examples, as well as Robin Lally, BA, BSN, RN for assistance with manuscript revision.

serves a chance. Therefore, she arranges a family meeting with both Sarah and Mary. During the meeting, Janet shares her observations and encourages Sarah and Mary to openly express their desires and concerns about the situation. After much discussion they reach a mutual decision that Sarah can try a 48-hour stay at her apartment. Mary will remain with her, but Sarah must carry out all activities as if Mary were not there. At the end of the trial period, Janet visits Sarah and Mary at the apartment. Sarah says that she now realizes, reluctantly, that she cannot stay alone and is willing to return to Sunnyvale. Janet and Mary feel pleased that Sarah has made her own decision about her living arrangements.

As this vignette illustrates, advanced practice nurses encounter patient situations that span time and setting. Such situations are often characterized by complexity, uncertainty, ambiguity, and/or instability (Lewis, 1997). In such situations, advanced practice nurses make autonomous as well as collaborative and interdisciplinary decisions. Also, they are called upon to assist others—e.g., nurses, patients, and families—as they make decisions. How do advanced practice nurses do all of this?

The focus of this chapter is on strategies that advanced practice nurses can use to: (a) enhance their own decision making about direct patient care; and (b) assist others, patients and families as well as other nurses, in making decisions about health care. Managerial and entrepreneurial decisions are excluded. In the next section, related literature is briefly summarized. Then five selected strategies are described and illustrated as they are used by advanced practice nurses in a variety of areas. The strategies are analogy, "thinking aloud," policy capturing, informal decision analysis, and paradigm case.

RELATED LITERATURE

Until recently, little has been known about *how* nurses make clinical decisions. "Nursing Process" was offered in the 1960s as the conceptualization of nurses' clinical reasoning; however, no research tested whether nurses actually used this process as described (Yura & Walsh, 1973). The introduction of "Nursing Process" was important in focusing on nurses as thinkers as well as doers, but it was limited in that it did not delineate either the underlying thinking processes or the specific knowledge involved.

In the 1960s, researchers began examining how nurses: (a) select relevant patient data from the large amount available in each situation, (b) combine this clinical data with their knowledge base to make inferences about the patient's status, and (c) choose appropriate interventions for a given situation (Corcoran & Tanner, 1988; Tanner, 1987). Although various theoretical perspectives on decision making were used in these studies, repeated findings documented that "Nursing Process" did not represent nurses' reasoning (Grobe, Drew, & Fonteyn, 1991; Tanner, 1987, 1988). Evidence indicated that nurses use an iterative (repetitive) approach to decision making involving both cognitive and intuitive processes, rather than the linear, purely cognitive approach suggested by "Nursing Process".

Initial research launched in the 1960s focused on describing nurses' analytical processes. Kenneth Hammond, a psychologist, collaborated with Katherine Kelly, a nurse, to study the clinical inferences made by nurses (Hammond, 1964, 1966; Hammond, Kelly, Schneider, & Vancini, 1966; Kelly, 1964). While they encountered methodological difficulties and had inconclusive findings, Hammond and colleagues' work was important in initiating research on this topic.

In the 1970s and 1980s, some nursing researchers shifted their focus to analytical processes that were prescriptive in nature. They pursued the congruity between nurses' natural decision making and a rational model of how decisions should be made. Grier (1976) used a decision-analytic perspective to study how nurses deliberated about alternative living arrangements for the elderly, action, the likely risks and benefits of each alternative in the given situation, and personal values related to potential outcomes of each option. She found that nurses were able to combine information to select actions that were consistent with their values and preferences, a process congruent with the rational model. Later, Baumann and Deber (1989) examined the limitations of a decision-analytic perspective for studying nurses' rapid decision making in the intensive care unit. However, Panniers and Walker (1994) found the decision-analytic process to be useful in nurses' clinical decision making about pressure ulcer dressing.

During this same period, other nursing researchers focused on describing how nurses process information when making clinical decisions. They became intrigued by two major assumptions of Information Processing Theory: (a) that human beings have a long-term memory with almost infinite capacity, and (b) their short-term memory (working memory) is limited to 7±2 "chunks" (a chunk is any organization of information that has previously become familiar) (Miller, 1956; Newell & Simon, 1972). Several research teams investigated how nurses processed information when collecting data to assess patients' conditions (Ellis, 1997; Tanner, Padrick, Westfall, & Putzier, 1987; White, Nativio, Kobert, & Engberg, 1992). They found that subjects used hypothetico-deductive reasoning to arrive at diagnoses. In this approach, subjects activated hypotheses early in the clinical situation based on minimal data and employed systematic data-gathering to test their hypotheses and form a diagnosis. Researchers interpreted subjects' use of hypothetico-deductive reasoning as a mechanism for dealing with their short-term memory limits in the face of large amounts of clinical data. These findings were consistent with Elstein, Shulman, and Sprafka's (1990) four-stage model of physicians' medical problem solving: problem sensing, hypothesis activation, data acquisition, and hypothesis evaluation.

Other nurse researchers using the information-processing perspective found that nurses, like other health professionals, use a range of analytical processes as well as a wealth of knowledge when making assessments and planning patient care (Corcoran, 1986b; Gordon, 1980; Grier, 1976; Grobe et al., 1991; Narayan & Corcoran-Perry, 1997; Tanner et al., 1987). Not surprisingly, these studies showed that the knowledge required was task-dependent; that is, different knowledge was needed for different decision-making tasks. Furthermore, investigators found that the processes, too, were task-dependent and iterative rather than linear.

Several investigations of nursing expertise compared the analytical reasoning of experienced nurses' (experts) with that of nurses new to an area of practice (novices). The novices served as a control so that the thinking processes of experts could be better understood. These studies revealed that experienced nurses were better than new nurses at: (a) collecting clinical data efficiently and understanding its significance; (b) recognizing the probabilistic relationship between data and patient conditions, as well as between nursing actions and patient outcomes; (c) accessing their knowledge, including both theoretical and practical (experience-based) knowledge; (d) generating more detailed and appropriate interventions; and (e) using general rules of thumb (heuristics) in their decision making (Corcoran, 1986b; Narayan & Corcoran-Perry, 1997; Tabak, Bar-Tal, & Cohen-Mansfield, 1996; Tanner et al., 1987).

Still other researchers investigated nurses' use of intuition. These researchers found that clinicians, particularly experienced nurses, used intuition as well as analytical processes to make clinical decisions. Intuition involves not only cognition, but also a sensory grasp of the whole situation within a particular context. (Benner, 1984; Benner, Tanner, &

Chesla, 1996; Rew, 1988). Benner and Tanner (1987) found that experienced nurses used six aspects of intuition: pattern recognition, similarity recognition, commonsense understanding, skilled know-how, sense of salience, and deliberative rationality. These aspects are developed through experiences with similar situations. For example, a nurse may walk into a patient's room and quickly recognize that "something is wrong." This nurse instantly recognizes a pattern observed previously in other patients or senses a change in this patient. This holistic grasp is in contrast to the analytical processes of attending to particular cues, combining the cues, and arriving at diagnostic inferences.

Since the late 1980s, more research has been directed at multiple aspects of individual and/or family caregiver's decision making about health care. For example, Pierce (1993) studied women's decision-making styles when choosing breast cancer surgical treatment. She found women using three different styles: deliberator, deferrer, and delayer. Owens, Ashcroft, Leinster, and Slade (1987) found an informal decision analysis approach to be effective when assisting women as they chose their breast cancer surgical treatment. When working with women who were making decisions about hormone replacement therapy, Rothert et al. (1997) found that multiple methods of providing relevant information were useful. Lewis, Pearson, Corcoran-Perry, and Narayan (1997) studied the nature and scope of decision-making situations encountered by family caregivers of persons with cancer.

SELECTED STRATEGIES

Analogy

An analogy is defined as "a resemblance in some particulars between things otherwise unlike, i.e., a similarity" (Jorgensen, 1980, p.2). Often an analogy is used to make the unfamiliar familiar, or to make the familiar unfamiliar (Alexander, White, Haensly, & Crimmins-Jeanes, 1987). It is a simple, but powerful, tool for developing both creative and critical thinking abilities. Consequently, analogies can be used to enhance both analytical and intuitive abilities.

The "synectic" model is a formal approach that incorporates analogies. It has five phases: (a) describe the present situation or problem; (b) present and describe an analogy for the situation; (c) describe the similarities between the analogy and the situation; (d) describe the differences between the analogy and the situation; and (e) re-explore the original situation on its own terms (Joyce, Weil, & Showers, 1992).

Advanced practice nurses often use analogies to simplify the mental image of a task, or to view a situation from another perspective. The following example illustrates how one public health nurse clinician, Ruth Abrams, used the Synectic Model to help new staff nurses develop a simple, but powerful mental representation.[1]

In team meetings, Ruth often heard new public health nurses describe patients in terms of their conditions. To counter this reductionistic perspective and to develop a sense of patients as whole indivisible persons, Ruth shared an analogy to represent holism. She began with Phase 1 in which she acknowledged the difficulty many people have grasping the concept of holism. She shared statements that she had heard which reflected this quandary.

In Phase 2, Ruth presented an analogy. She began by setting on the table jars of flour, milk, sugar, butter, eggs, and baking powder. She asked, "What do I have here?" The nurses listed the ingredients. Then Ruth took all the ingredients out of the jars, put them into a bowl, mixed them together and asked, "What do I have now?" The nurses indicated a mixture of ingredients. The next question was, "Can I retrieve any of the individual ingredients?" to which the answer was "No." Next Ruth said, "Imagine that I have put these mixed ingredients into a pan and placed them in an oven at 350 degrees for one hour. Here is what I have," as she revealed a cake. Then Ruth asked the nurses to describe the analogy. The nurses stated: "We ended up with something very different from the ingredients with which we began, a cake;" "The separate ingredients to make the cake are not visible;" "The ingredients cannot be pulled out;" and "A transformation occurred in the ingredients as they were mixed and heated." This phase helped nurses gain insight into the meaning of the term, "whole." They came to view the "whole" of a cake as something greater than and different from the sum of its ingredients. Their creative abilities were promoted as they visualized the ingredients being combined and taking on a new identity.

In Phase 3, Ruth asked the nurses to describe the similarities between the cake and a whole person. The nurses repeated the statements about the inability to distinguish or extract the parts, whether of a cake or a

---

[1]This example is a modification of one presented in Corcoran & Tanner, 1988.

person. They talked about both the cake and a person being greater than and different from the sum of the parts. They concluded that persons are more than their physical, psychological, social, and spiritual parts. The nurses also indicated that one could examine the parts, for example, the quality of the flour or the quality of a person's heart; and that the quality of the parts could influence the quality of the whole, but did not describe the whole.

In Phase 4, Ruth asked the nurses to focus on the differences between a cake and a person. They identified the primary differences between the nature of a cake as an inanimate object and of a person as a living, dynamic being. Then they explored these differences in greater detail.

In Phase 5, Ruth and the nurses re-examined the concept of holism. For example, they explored the language that would represent a view of persons as holistic beings. After completing this activity, they reflected on the thinking processes they had used in working with the analogy.

As indicated earlier, analogies can be used to promote both creative and critical thinking, two processes central to nurses' clinical decision making. Creative thinking abilities are relevant to intuitive processes such as pattern recognition, similarity recognition, and commonsense understanding (Benner & Tanner, 1987). For example, analogies can help one relate a familiar past experience to a seemingly unfamiliar current situation. Creativity is also relevant to analytical processes such as hypothesis generation during diagnostic reasoning and the generation of possible interventions when planning nursing care. For example, analogies can help one visualize multiple interpretations of cues or causes of a patient's presenting symptoms. Similarly, analogies can stimulate thinking about multiple and innovative ways for dealing with a given situation.

"Thinking Aloud"

"Thinking aloud" is a strategy for enhancing analytical abilities. Originally, "thinking aloud" was used as a data collection method in research on the cognitive processes people use to solve problems or make decisions. While the intent of this research was to understand how experts thought and to help others think accordingly, experts were usually unable to describe how they performed tasks (Johnson, 1983). One way that researchers overcame this paradox was to have experts "think aloud" while actually performing a particular task. Corcoran, Narayan, and

Moreland (1988) proposed that this strategy also would be useful for developing nurses' skill in decision making.

When implementing this strategy, a clinician "thinks aloud" while making a decision about a specific clinical situation (either real or hypothetical). The "thinking aloud" verbalizations may be tape recorded and later transcribed. The recordings or transcripts can be analyzed for such aspects as the data to which the clinician attends, the way data are clustered, the knowledge used, the hypotheses activated, and the rules of thumb employed to combine information and make decisions.

"Thinking aloud" is illustrated with an excerpt of the transcript from an orthopaedic clinical nurse specialist, Eric Olson.[2] As part of his quality assurance responsibilities, Eric regularly meets with his clinical specialist colleagues to examine potential nursing care problems. Eric is to present an issue at the next meeting. Recently he noted that several orthopaedic patients had developed severe cardiac complications following surgery. He wonders whether the staff nurses are recognizing early indicators of these complications. Are they detecting and intervening soon enough? He decides to tape record and transcribe his "thinking aloud" comments as he reviews the chart of one patient who experienced such a complication.

At the meeting with the clinical nurses, Eric shares the transcript of his chart review. (See Table 5.1 for the transcription.) After initial review of the transcript, the group concludes that the nurses involved should have detected a potential problem earlier and could have intervened sooner. Then they analyze the excerpt further to discover what the nurses may have missed. The group notes that Eric attended to the patient's age, complexity and length of surgery, and medications as critical cues. He interpreted that these factors would predispose the patient to complications, particularly cardiac and fluid problems. His awareness of these potential problems guided his subsequent focus on intake and output data, as well as vital signs. Group members speculate that the nurses working with this patient may have overlooked the critical cues and/or failed to cluster the cues as Eric did, particularly since the patient's medical history did not emphasize cardiac conditions.

According to the transcript, Eric determined that the patient's output was much lower than his intake on the day of surgery. However, the nurses working with the patient apparently did not detect this discrepancy that day, because they did not notify the physician until the next day. Eric recalls hearing orthopaedic nurses frequently say: "Our patients almost always have low urine volumes postoperatively." He speculates

---

[2]This example was first presented in Corcoran-Perry and Bungert (1992).

TABLE 5.1   Excerpt of "Thinking Aloud" Transcript

I want to identify information the nurses had available to them at the time indicating that this patient was developing problems. Should we have intervened sooner?

Here it indicates that the patient was a 74-year-old male.

The OR report has a very lengthy description of a decompression laminectomy at L4-5, L5-S1. He went into surgery at 11:45, came out at 16:08, and spent 4 hours in the recovery room.

This tells me that the patient had a complicated procedure and was in the OR for a long time. These factors would predispose him to problems.

The next thing I am looking at is the patient's past history. Is he predisposed to cardiac problems? This is important because people over 65 tend to have chronic diseases for which they take a minimum of five medications. ·

The nurse's admission notes indicate a history of hypertension. The medical history notes indicates hypertension and a questionable MI.

The list of medications seems to indicate a much more complicated medical history than is stated. He has been on Naprosyn, Lopressor, Allopurinol, Lanoxin, Lasix, Hydrocholorthiazide, and extra-strength Tylenol. The Tylenol and Naprosyn could indeed be for conditions related to his surgery. The Lopressor is for his hypertension, but the Lanoxin suggests cardiac problems. Lasix and Hydrochlorothiazide, both diuretics, indicate fluid problems.

So, this information alerts me to watch this patient postoperatively for his output, particularly with the length of surgery and the amount of fluids he would get.

So I want to look at trends in his intake, output, and vital signs.

On the day of surgery, he received 4000 cc. of IV fluids and 250 cc. orally. So, his total intake was 4250 cc. He had an estimated blood loss of 1000 cc, drainage of 50 cc., and urine output of 575 cc. His Foley catheter was irrigated and apparently open. So, his output is much lower than his intake. On his first post-op day his output is described as "80 cc. of very dark, concentrated urine." The physician was notified.

Immediately post-op, his blood pressure was 144/100, his pulse 80, and his respirations 18. His breath sounds were described as diminished with some SOB and he was given oxygen.

On the first post-op day, his respirations increased to 24–28. His pulse was recorded as 100 and irregular. His blood pressure varied markedly. It was 120/70 at midnight, 180/90 at 8:00, and 104/84 at 16:00.

In the evening of the first post-op day, the physician ordered Lasix. It was given IV at 16:40. Now I'm looking for information about his response to the Lasix. It could start having an effect at 20 minutes, but possibly up to an hour. But no indication of response at 20:00 when his BP dropped to 76/60. The physician was called regarding the low blood pressure, shortness of breath, thready pulse, and low urine output. He was put on a monitor and transferred to the critical care unit late morning the second post-op day.

Note: From "Enhancing Orthopaedic Nurses' Clinical Decision Making" by S. A. Corcoran-Perry, & B. Bungert (1992). *Orthopaedic Nursing, 11,* p. 68. Copyright 1992 by Corcoran-Perry. Reprinted with permission.

that because of this perception, the nurses probably do not interpret low urine volume as unusual or critical. He does not know their basis for this statement, nor how "low" is quantified.

One member of the group identifies that the nurse(s) involved in this situation seem to be operating on a simple rule of thumb: "Low urine volume is a common benign occurrence in orthopaedic patients postoperatively." The group suggests that nurses on the orthopaedic unit measure patients' postoperative urine volumes over time and document related outcomes. Then the nurses will have specific information about what constitutes "low" urine volume and the nature of related outcomes. The cardiovascular clinical specialist offers to conduct a staff development session on the additional monitoring needed for persons who have or might develop cardiovascular conditions when they undergo surgery.

One of the group members indicates that she would like to reflect on the hypothetico-deductive approach that Eric used. She points out that Eric generated an early hypothesis (predisposition to complications) based on minimal cues (age, complexity and length of surgery, and medication). Also, he used this hypothesis to guide further data collection (focusing on vital signs and fluid balance trends). She suggests that nurses on the unit would benefit from this kind of "thinking aloud" approach. Their verbalizations would enable them to acquire a better understanding of their decision-making processes, appreciate the richness of their clinical knowledge, improve their clinical reasoning by linking the knowledge and processes used to specific patient outcomes, and reveal underlying causes of errors in clinical reasoning. Such errors may be revealed through feedback from peers or experts.

All members of the clinical specialist group indicate that "thinking aloud" is very helpful. This experience gave them an opportunity to reflect on the clinical judgments made, as well as the feelings generated and actions taken within a particular context. Even though the knowledge that they gained could not change what happened in this situation, they appreciate that their insights can influence their future reasoning and actions in similar situations.

Policy Capturing

When much information is available for decision making, it is difficult to know which data are important and how to combine them. Social Judgment Theory focuses on describing how humans make decisions under conditions of uncertainty (Cooksey, 1996; Elstein & Bordage, 1979). Policy capturing is one method associated with this theory that reveals how people weigh and combine information. It is a strategy that identifies the selected factors that persons take into account when making a judgment and the relative weights they assign to the factors. Once a policy is captured and represented, often in the form of a formula, it can be used to communicate and/or justify an analytical judgment.

Policy capturing is illustrated in the following situation. Alicia Hernandez, an advanced practice nurse, is serving as a nursing representative to an interdisciplinary expert panel convened by the State Department of Health. The panel is charged with developing recommendations about the necessity for and appropriateness of practice restrictions for human immunodeficiency virus (HIV)-infected health professionals. The panel is challenged to make recommendations that protect the public by providing safe health care and that respect infected health professionals' rights to privacy and nondiscrimination in employment. Three policy options are to be considered: (a) mandatory practice restrictions of infected health professionals in performance of exposure-prone, invasive procedures; (b) voluntary practice restrictions, in which infected health professionals are educated and encouraged to restrict their own practice of exposure-prone procedures; and (c) no practice restrictions.

The panel members review the extensive material and spend hours discussing the options and their implications. They seem to go over the same information repeatedly. Alicia suggests that they try a policy-capturing strategy which may help them identify and weigh factors that are important in considering practice restrictions for HIV-infected health professionals. The group agrees to try the strategy.

Upon reflection, panel members realize that they consistently focus on four factors: HIV infection rate, the route of transmission, and the possible consequences for patients as well as those for health care workers. This helps narrow their focus of attention. Next they individually assign weights (beginning with low, medium, or high weights) to each factor. The weights represent the contribution of each factor to their consideration of restricting practice.

All panel members report assigning a low weight to HIV infection rate. Since the infection rate is low, it is not a major contributor to a decision to restrict practice. Similarly, most panel members reveal that they assigned a high weight to possible consequences for patients, since it is believed that all HIV-infected persons will eventually die. Most members assigned moderate weights to the two remaining factors, route of HIV transmission and consequences for the health professionals. At this stage Alicia develops the following formula as a representation of their emerging policy:

Restriction Policy = low wt.(a) + high wt.(b) + mod. wt(c) + mod. wt.(d) + C

Note: a = infection rate
            b = consequences for patients
            c = routes of transmission
            d = consequences for health professionals
            C = constant or error term

Panel members identify that the policy-capturing process is useful in emphasizing the factors that they consider to be most important. Also, they feel reassured that they independently assigned similar weights to each factor and, therefore, that some type of practice restriction is needed.

When examining the formula, panel members recognize that although they all assigned moderate weights to the last two factors, they feel uneasy about them. Members report that "route of transmission" and "consequence for health professionals" are difficult to conceptualize. They reflect that the limited routes of HIV transmission restrict the possibilities for transmitting the disease in most circumstances, but that the invasive procedures conducted by some health professionals increase the chances of infection. This implies variability according to health care discipline, procedure, and technique. Regarding possible consequences for the infected health professional, the panel members identify that health professionals could suffer multiple harms from having their practice restricted, including social, economic, professional, and psychological harms. For example, their HIV-infected status could easily be revealed to persons who have no right or need to know about it. Consequently, the panel members decide that they need to do further work in explicating the multidimensional aspects of these two factors. Therefore, each member will gather relevant information specific to their discipline and various areas of practice to share with the group.

The strategy of policy capturing provides not only a model for representing thought and judgment, but also a mechanism for promoting communication. As Engel, Wigton, LaDuca, and Blacklow (1990) point out:

> when communication about the policy model is centered on the model as metaphor, attention is focused on the exchange of ideas about knowledge and relationships. This arrangement breaks down traditional role boundaries, makes each person an active participant, and fosters a collaborative and constructive relationship between (professionals) (p. 75).

Informal Decision Analysis

Decision analysis, a methodology for choosing among mutually exclusive options, provides a mechanism for promoting rational decision making. It provides both a structure and procedure that enables decision makers to choose actions that are consistent with what they know and value (Corcoran, 1986a; Elstein & Bordage, 1979; Raiffa, 1968). Decision analysis may be either formal or informal. Formal decision analysis involves a mathematical procedure for prescribing the best option; that is, the one most consistent with what is known and valued. This formal approach is described in detail elsewhere (Corcoran, 1986a; Raiffa, 1968).

Informal decision analysis involves a non-mathematical approach to decision making, while still incorporating the basic concepts of formal decision analysis. The structure consists of four major components: (a) options, (b) possible outcomes, (c) values assigned to the outcomes, and (d) likelihoods that the options will lead to the outcomes. The procedure is less technical than formal decision analysis in that mathematical calculations are not used. Instead, the decision maker is guided to conceptually consider and combine information.

The *OOVL Decision-making Guide* (Lewis, Hepburn, Corcoran-Perry, Narayan, & Lally (1998) is one tool based on informal decision analysis that advanced practice nurses can use to enhance their own clinical decision making and to support patients and families when making choices. As with other forms of informal decision analysis, the *OOVL Guide* provides decision makers with both a structure and a procedure. The structure is in the form of a grid representing options, outcomes, values, and likelihoods (see Figure 5.1). In addition, a series of questions guide the person through the decision-making process. Informal decision analysis using the *OOVL Decision-making Guide* is illustrated by the following scenario.

During a support group for spouses of patients at a Veteran's Hospital Alzheimer's clinic, Agnes Embers describes her situation. She lives with her husband, Lloyd, a 75-year-old with Dementia, Alzheimer's Type. Lloyd was diagnosed 1 year ago. In the last 6 months, Agnes has noticed an increase in his short-term memory loss. For example, when they drive to the grocery store, he asks her which way to turn. Lloyd has always been the driver in the family; Agnes never learned to drive. They drive primarily on neighborhood streets during daylight hours, and Lloyd drives to breakfast with friends every Thursday. Agnes expresses concern about Lloyd's driving. She knows he will not voluntarily give up driving, and therefore, she must decide if she should take the car keys away from him.

The support group helps Agnes work through the *OOVL Decision Making Guide* using the following questions:

1. What do you need to make a decision about? Agnes again indicates that she wants to decide what to do about her husband's driving. (Figure 5.1 depicts a completed *OOVL Decision-making Guide* for this decision.)

2. What actions are you considering? Agnes considers three options: (a) Lloyd continues driving alone; (b) Agnes limits his driving to when they are together; and (c) Agnes takes the car keys away from Lloyd.

3. What would you like to have happen as a result of your choice? Whatever option is chosen, there will be consequences. Agnes considers what she would like to have occur, as well as what she hopes to avoid happening. The four outcomes that she identifies are: (a) safety for themselves and others; (b) their ability to come and go freely; (c) preserving Lloyd's self-respect; and (d) avoiding marital discord (e.g., the two of them arguing over his driving).

4. How important is each of these outcomes to you? The importance of the outcomes may be identified by placing values on them. Positive outcomes can be assigned + signs, and negative values are given – signs.

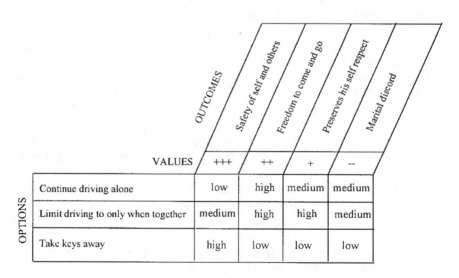

OPTIONS	OUTCOMES / VALUES	Safety of self and others / +++	Freedom to come and go / ++	Preserves his self respect / +	Marital discord / --
	Continue driving alone	low	high	medium	medium
	Limit driving to only when together	medium	high	high	medium
	Take keys away	high	low	low	low

FIGURE 5.1   *OOVL* Grid for Driving Decision

The more important outcomes can be assigned a greater number of + or – signs. Another way to represent the values is to rank-order the outcomes. Agnes assigns the following values to each outcome: (a) safety (+++); (b) ability to come and go freely (++); (c) preserving Lloyd's self-respect (+); and (4) avoiding marital discord (–).

5. How likely or possible is it that each option will lead to each of the outcomes? The decision maker must consider the likelihood that the option will lead to the outcomes. The advanced practice nurse may provide information, if data are available; however, the person's personal experience is the primary source of information about the likelihood that an option will achieve an outcome. In informal decision analysis, words, instead of probability values, are used to represent likelihoods. Agnes rates each likelihood as high, medium, or low. (See Figure 5.1 for the completed decision grid.) for the likelihoods that she assigned to each outcome for each option.

6. What option is most likely to achieve the best outcomes? Although the grid serves as a guide in the decision-making process, the person must relate the information about each option, and compare the options. Agnes quickly eliminates the first option (Lloyd continues driving alone), because of her concern for safety, and the medium likelihood that he will have reduced self-respect. Also, because of his short-term memory loss, he is likely to get lost if he drives alone. In comparing the second and third options (limit Lloyd's driving and taking away the car keys), Agnes decides that the second option, limiting Lloyd's driving to when they are together, has the best likelihood of accomplishing the desired outcomes and minimizing the negative outcome of marital discord. Agnes and the other members of the support group found the *OOVL Decision-making Guide* to be very helpful. They recognized that different people may identify other options and outcomes, and assign different values and likelihoods because of their individual values and preferences.

Although less complex than formal decision analysis, completing the informal decision-making grid does require time and energy to reflect about the components of the decision. Therefore, it is particularly suitable for serious and complex decisions, and those for which there is adequate time for deliberation.

In addition to promoting rational choice, informal decision analysis can be useful in pinpointing the basis for differing judgments between professional colleagues, family members, or patients and professionals. For example, a decision analysis grid may reveal varying interpretations or valuing of outcomes that lead to different judgments.

Paradigm Cases

Benner was the first nurse researcher to report using paradigm cases to study nurses' lived experiences in clinical practice (Benner, 1984; Benner & Tanner, 1987). A paradigm case is a narrative description of a past instance that stands out in a nurse's memory, e.g., a situation in which the nurse's decisions and/or actions made a difference, either positively or negatively. Such a case is repeatedly called to mind. By sharing a paradigm case with colleagues, all may gain new knowledge that comes only from experience or transform old knowledge. Table 5.2 contains an excerpt from one advanced practice nurse's paradigm case told as a story to a group of experienced colleagues.

The group members reflected on Kathy's paradigm case and were

TABLE 5.2   Excerpt of a Paradigm Case

One patient I often think of is Helen, an older lady that I worked with for several years. She was a severe diabetic with many problems. She had the worst feet I'd ever seen, "classic diabetic feet"—bad arches, big fat feet that looked like boxes. You would touch the skin and she'd get a big ulcer. She needed a nurse and good chronic care. Prior to the time that I worked with her she was hospitalized about every 3 months with major sepsis. I started seeing her in clinic, and we worked together on her foot care for years. Her mobility was important to her, even if she couldn't get around very well. She was willing to try anything to be able to walk and stay out of the hospital.

What really seemed to help was getting her into Unna Boots. I'd see her weekly and change the boots. I could see if infection was starting and treat her with antibiotics right away. The boots really seemed to help—although her feet never looked normal. We kept her out of the hospital for about 5 years. Then an enterostomal therapist joined our staff. So I referred Helen to her. I continued to see Helen for her diabetes, but didn't go with her to the enterostomal therapist after the initial session. Several months later I saw Helen and didn't think her feet looked so good. I talked with the therapist and she said they were having some problems. I suggested that Helen see the foot specialist in the diabetic clinic. The next thing I knew, they admitted her to the hospital and had her seen by a vascular surgeon who threatened an amputation. I was shocked! I immediately went to see Helen in her hospital room. When I looked at her left foot it looked bad, but certainly no worse than when I was seeing her in clinic. I just hit the roof. Right away I called the enterostomal therapist and the surgeon. I demanded that the surgeon come and examine her foot with me. I really raised a fuss and would not take "No" for an answer. The surgeon did come and examine Helen's foot with me. After I told him of my longstanding care of Helen and our success with the Unna Boot, he agreed that superficial debridement was called for, and not an amputation.

surprised at the number of clinical decisions inherent in her account, e.g., diagnosing significant changes in Helen's feet, choosing Unna boots to prevent infection, selecting antibiotics when infections occurred, judging when referrals were appropriate, and determining how best to serve as Helen's advocate. Members were struck by how the quality of Kathy's decisions was influenced by her knowledge of Helen's particular responses and circumstances, based on the many years in which she had worked with her. One nurse emphasized how "knowing the patient" is central to skilled clinical judgment "Knowing the patient" involves both recognizing and understanding the patient's typical pattern, as well as knowing the patient as a person (Tanner, Benner, Chesla, & Gordon, 1993). Recognition and understanding of the patient's typical pattern was evident in Kathy's story as she described the appearance of Helen's feet over time, detecting changes that occurred, and interpreting whether such changes warranted treatment. Knowing the patient as a person was apparent in Kathy's interpretation of the impact of an amputation on Helen's life. The group indicated that the power of this story was that it triggered recall of their own experiences in which "knowing the patient" really made a difference. This special kind of knowledge and resulting commitment to the patient involved actions linked directly to patient outcomes. Sharing these experiences highlighted the importance of continuity of care, accentuating the role played by advanced practice nurses. The group decided that sharing similar stories about their experiences could lead to delineation and elaboration of significant, but little understood aspects of clinical decision making.

SUMMARY

Research findings indicate that nurses, like other health professionals, use a wide range of analytical and intuitive processes during clinical decision making (Benner et al., 1996; Corcoran, 1986a, 1986b; Tanner, 1987). Since no strategy addresses all aspects of decision making, we selected five strategies that advanced practice nurses can use to enhance their own decision making and that of others. The strategies are: analogy, "thinking aloud," policy capturing, informal decision analysis, and paradigm cases. Now that each of these strategies has been described and illustrated, we will highlight some important distinctions.

Two of the strategies, analogies and paradigm cases, are more useful for gaining an overall grasp of a situation than are the other strategies. An analogy helps one view a situation from a different perspective, while a paradigm case teaches a lesson through a particular and powerful story. Because the other strategies—thinking aloud, policy capturing, and informal decision analysis—emphasize components of decision making, they are helpful in strengthening particular skills. For example, "thinking aloud" and policy-capturing strategies reveal the information to which a decision maker attends and the way data are clustered or combined.

Time is another element that differentiates potential uses of the strategies. If the intent is to understand the actual decision making processes used, then it is important that the strategy be concurrent with the person's decision making. For example, asking an advanced practice nurse to "think aloud" *while* making a decision is likely to reveal her/his underlying cognitive processes and heuristics. However, if the nurse is asked to describe how she/he usually makes a certain type of decision, she/he is apt to reconstruct a plausible explanation. In contrast, policy capturing does not need to be concurrent with the person's decision making. The intent of this strategy is to develop a representation that performs like an individual does, but the representation is not of the person's actual information-processing. Policy capturing is more relevant to group decision making than are the other strategies. Generally, the development of a policy is a group activity, while "thinking aloud" is an individual endeavor.

The analytical and intuitive processes examined here are necessary components of decision making, but by no means sufficient. Obviously, decision making about health care requires an accurate and current knowledge base. We are reminded of the analogy: Knowledge is to decision making as sin is to confession; without the first, there is nothing to say in the second.

REFERENCES

Alexander, P., White, C., Haensly, P., & Crimmins-Jeanes, M. (1987). Training in analogical reasoning. *American Educational Research Journal, 24,* 387–404.

Baumann, A., & Deber, R. (1989). The limits of decision analysis for rapid decision making in ICU nursing. *IMAGE: Journal of Nursing Scholarship, 21,* 69–71.

Benner, P. (1984). *From novice to expert: Excellence and power in clinical nursing practice.* Menlo Park, CA: Addison-Wesley.

Benner, P., & Tanner, C. (1987). Clinical judgment: How expert nurses use intuition. *American Journal of Nursing, 87,* 23–31.

Benner, P. A., Tanner, C. A., & Chesla, C. A. (1996). *Expertise in nursing practice: Caring, clinical judgment, and ethics.* New York: Springer.

Cooksey, R. (1996). *Judgment analysis: Theory, methods, and applications.* San Diego, CA: Academic Press.

Corcoran, S. (1986a). Decision analysis: A step-by-step guide for making clinical decisions. *Nursing and Health Care, 7,* 149–154.

Corcoran, S. (1986b). Task complexity and nursing expertise as factors in decision making. *Nursing Research, 35,* 107–112.

Corcoran, S., Narayan, S., & Moreland, H. (1988). Thinking aloud as a strategy to improve clinical decision making. *Heart & Lung, 17,* 463–468.

Corcoran, S., & Tanner, C. (1988). Implications of judgment research for teaching. In *Curriculum revolution: Mandate for change* (pp. 159–176). New York: National League for Nursing.

Corcoran-Perry, S., & Bungert, B. (1992). Enhancing orthopaedic nurses' clinical decision making. *Orthopaedic Nursing, 11*(3), 64–70.

Ellis, P. (1997). Processes used by nurses to make decisions in the clinical practice setting. *Nurse Education Today, 17,* 325–332.

Elstein, A., & Bordage, G. (1979). Psychology of clinical reasoning. In G. Stone, F. Cohen, & N. Alder (Eds.). *Health psychology* (pp. 333–367). San Francisco: Jossey-Bass.

Elstein, A., Shulman, L., & Sprafka, S. (1990). Medical problem solving: A ten-year retrospective. *Evaluation & the Health Professions, 13,* 5–36.

Engel, J., Wigton, R., LaDuca, A., & Blacklow, R. (1990). A Social Judgment Theory perspective on clinical problem solving. *Evaluation and the Health Professions, 13,* 63–78.

Gordon, M. (1980). Predictive strategies in diagnostic tasks. *Nursing Research, 29,* 39–45

Grier, M. (1976). Decision making about patient care. *Nursing Research, 25,* 105–110.

Grobe, S., Drew, J., & Fonteyn, M. (1991). A descriptive analysis of experienced nurses' clinical reasoning during a planning task. *Research in Nursing and Health, 14,* 305–324.

Hammond, K. (1964). Clinical inference in nursing: A methodological approach. *Nursing Research, 13,* 315–319.

Hammond, K. (1966). Clinical inference in nursing: A psychologist's viewpoint. *Nursing Research, 15,* 27–38.

Hammond, K., Kelly, K., Schneider, R., & Vancini, M. (1966). Clinical inference in nursing: Analyzing cognitive tasks representative of nursing problems. *Nursing Research, 15,* 134–138.

Kelly, K. (1964). An approach to the study of clinical inference in nursing: Part III. Utilization of the "Lens Model" method to study the inferential process of the nurse. *Nursing Research, 13,* 319–322.

Johnson, P. (1983). What kind of expert should a system be? *Journal of Medicine and Philosophy, 8,* 77–97.

Jorgensen, S. (1980). *Using analogies to develop conceptual abilities.* (ERIC Reports, #ED 192 820). Washington, DC: U.S. Department of Health, Education, and Welfare, National Institute of Education.

Joyce, B., Weil, M., & Showers, B. (1992). *Models of teaching* (4th ed.). Boston: Allyn & Bacon.

Lewis, M. (1997). Decision making task complexity: Model development and initial testing. *Journal of Nursing Education, 36,* 114–120.

Lewis, M., Hepburn, K., Corcoran-Perry, S., Narayan, S., & Lally, R. (1998). *OOVL Decision-making guide for patients and families.* Manuscript submitted for publication, University of Minnesota.

Lewis, M., Pearson, V., Corcoran-Perry, S., & Narayan, S. (1997). Decision making by elderly patients with cancer and their caregivers. *Cancer Nursing, 20,* 389–397.

Miller, G. (1956). The magical number seven, plus or minus two. *Psychological Review, 63,* 81–87.

Narayan, S., & Corcoran-Perry, S. (1997). Line of reasoning as a representation of nurses' clinical decision making. *Research in Nursing and Health, 20,* 353–364.

Newell, A., & Simon, H. (1972). *Human problem solving.* Englewood Cliffs, NJ: Prentice-Hall.

Owens, R., Ashcroft, J., Leinster, S., & Slade, P. (1987). Informal decision analysis with breast cancer patients; An aid to psychological preparation for surgery. *Journal of Psychosocial Oncology, 5,* 23–33.

Panniers, T., & Walker, E. (1994). A decision-analytic approach to clinical nursing. *Nursing Research 43,* 245–249.

Pierce, P. (1993). Deciding on breast cancer treatment: A description of decision behavior. *Nursing Research, 42,* 22–28.

Raiffa, H. (1968). *Decision analysis: Introductory lectures on choice under uncertainty.* Menlo Park, CA. Addison Wesley.

Rew, L. (1988). Intuition in decision-making. *Image: The Journal of Nursing Scholarship, 20,* 150–154.

Rothert, M. L., Holmes-Rovner, M., Rovner, D., Kroll, J., Breer, L., Talarczyk, G., Schmitt, N., Padonu, G., & Wills, C. E. (1997). An educational intervention as decision support for menopausal women. *Research in Nursing & Health, 20,* 377–387.

Tabak, N., Bar-Tal, Y., & Cohen-Mansfield, J. (1996). Clinical decision making of experienced and novice nurses. *Western Journal of Nursing Research, 18,* 534–547.

Tanner, C. (1987). Teaching clinical judgment. In J. Fitzpatrick & R. Taunton (Eds.), *Annual Review of Nursing Research* (Vol. 5, pp. 153–173). New York: Springer Publishing Company.

Tanner, C. (1988). Curriculum revolution: The practice mandate. *Nursing and Health Care, 9,* 427–430.

Tanner, C., Benner, P., Chesla, C., & Gordon, D. (1993). The phenomenology of knowing the patient. *Image: Journal of Nursing Scholarship, 25,* 273–280.

Tanner, C., Padrick, K., Westfall, U., & Putzier, D. (1987). Diagnostic reasoning strategies of nurses and nursing students. *Nursing Research, 36,* 358–363.

White, J., Nativio, D., Kobert, S., & Engberg, S. (1992). Content and process in clinical decision-making by nurse practitioners. *Image: Journal of Nursing Scholarship, 24,* 153–158.

Yura, H., & Walsh, M. (1973). *The nursing process.* New York: Appleton.

Chapter 6

APN CARE MANAGERS AND CARE PATHWAYS

Kathleen Krichbaum, RN, PhD

Mr. H is an 81-year-old retired, married man who lives in a small home in a large city with his wife of 57 years. He had polio as a child and uses a walker to get around in his house. A few months ago, while going to the bathroom, he fell and fractured his left hip. He was admitted to a large suburban hospital and had surgery that day to repair the hip. Three days later, he was discharged to a transitional care unit in a local nursing home for 2 to 3 weeks of rehabilitation. His stay extended to 1 month due to his developing clinical depression that affected his motivation to attend physical therapy sessions. He developed a urinary tract infection and was placed on antibiotics. His wife came to visit every day, as did his two children, who were occasionally accompanied by their spouses. Mr. H's goal was to get back home and to have his life return to "normal." However, he found himself alone and lonely much of the time.

The staff at the nursing home was pleasant, even though it seemed as if there were not enough of them to answer his call light very quickly. He often had to wait to go to the bathroom. During his third week in the nursing home, there was a team conference held to plan for discharge of Mr. H. This conference was attended by his nurses, physical therapists, occupational therapists, social worker, the medical director, and a clinical psychologist. Mr. H was discussed; the plan was to have the psychologist see him and for the doctor to reassess his UTI. He would be discharged as soon as the depression and UTI were resolved.

Mr. H is typical of many elders who have experienced a traumatic event that places them squarely at the heart of the health care delivery system. Patients are treated for the immediate problem and released in a short time to figure out what to do—sometimes with a home caregiver to help, and sometimes without. Although Mr. H is elderly, his experience is one that might mirror that of any client, regardless of age or disease or injury. What about his experience is typical? Why are so many of his needs going unrecognized and unmet, despite the involvement of so many professionals? The questions raised speak to the nature of the current health care system. The solutions can be found in the response of nurses to the questions. This chapter will address the current climate experienced by clients in the health care delivery system as exemplified by Mr. H, and will explore the use of pathways and care management by advanced practice nurses as a thoughtful and appropriate response. Although the example of Mr. H is taken from the practice of APNs in gerontology, the solutions are applicable across populations and settings. The problems we face as APNs in meeting clients needs is universal.

THE CHANGING WORLD OF HEALTH CARE: HOW ARE WE MANAGING?

The American health care delivery system is undergoing fundamental change. It is being reconfigured into a system of managed care. "Managed care" essentially is an organized approach to coordinating or overseeing the care delivered to enrolled populations in order to achieve "some combination of cost reduction, enhanced patient and consumer satisfaction, and improvement of health care outcomes "(Pew Health Professions Commission, 1995). This revised approach to health care delivery is based on principles of efficiency (reducing costs), and effectiveness assessed in terms of achievement of outcomes that include both general outcomes (satisfaction) and outcomes specific to the population served (e.g., more functional independence for Mr. H following his hip fracture). It was proposed as a solution to the burgeoning costs associated with health care delivery in the United States realized since Medicare was passed into law in 1965. Managed care has been touted as a means to improve the quality of the health care delivery system as well. It is based on the philosophical notions put forth by W. Edward Deming and others that have come to be known as Total Quality Management or Continuous Quality Improvement. These approaches center on analyzing the processes used to manufacture a product or deliver a service (Deming, 1989).

In theory, one can improve both the efficiency and effectiveness of production of goods or services by carefully defining the processes used and then by monitoring adherence to those processes. Variances from what is defined hold the answers to inefficiencies. Explaining the variance and correcting the cause will lead to knowledge about the "best way to do things". The process can be corrected in order to increase productivity. This approach makes good fiscal sense; however, whether or not it is the most effective way to produce good client outcomes in health care certainly depends on how those outcomes are defined. The outcome of better health and better quality of life for their clients, for which APNs strive, is not necessarily achieved solely by the efficient use of resources.

CRITICAL PATHWAYS: THE TOOLS TO MANAGE CARE

A direct result of the interest in care outcomes for clients and in defining the processes of care is the emergence of an array of techniques and tools that are being used to describe those processes and their impact on outcomes in clients. There has occurred a parallel increase in empirical studies that seek to examine the effectiveness of these tools and techniques. One of the most popular tools is the critical pathway.

As discussed earlier, in order to manage care more effectively, one must first define the process or processes used to produce the outcome. In health care, the move to define the processes of care (including medical and nursing interventions), has taken the form of developing critical pathways (CP). Other descriptors like protocols or guidelines have been used to define what are essentially a set of standardized processes, critical interventions sequenced to move the client toward the outcomes that are predetermined to signal success for a given condition within a given time frame (Marschke & Nolan, 1993). The processes defined consist of actions to be taken by various caregivers that produce outcomes, or resulting client states or conditions that can be observed to measure success.

Most activity in the development of pathways has occurred in acute care where nursing has been the chief contributor. However, in recent years, the concept of pathways has been adopted in various settings from nursing homes and long-term care facilities (Riley, 1994) to home care agencies (Gartner & Twardon, 1995). Professionals in each of these various settings have developed pathways that define the processes of care to be used to treat clients with specific diagnoses within that setting. The pathways are, therefore, unique to that setting, and encompass the client's projected stay there.

Critical Pathways (CP) define "the optimal sequencing and timing of interventions by physicians, nurses and other staff for a particular diagnosis or procedure, designed to better utilize resources, maximize quality of care and minimize delays" (Coffey et al., 1992, p.46). As tools that are integral to managing care effectively, CPs have been investigated in terms of certain outcomes in acute care. Benefits of CPs include reduced length of stay (LOS) for clients with myocardial infarction (Etheredge, 1989), for cardiac transplantation hospitalization (Noedel et al., 1996), for coronary artery bypass graft patients in terms of hospital and surgical length of stay, for ischemic stroke patients in intensive care unit days (Zander, 1988), for cesarean section patients (Cohen, 1991), for radical prostatectomy (Koch & Smith, 1996), for lower extremity amputation (Schaldach, 1997), and others (Ethridge & Lamb, 1989; Zander, 1988). Mabrey and colleagues (1998) demonstrated reduced length of stay and reduced costs in patients having total knee arthroplasty. Other studies reported a reduction in costs and charges associated with use of CPs to guide care (Cohen, 1991; Koch & Smith, 1996; Zander, 1988).

In a study of the use of pathways used in critical care to produce earlier weaning of patients on long-term mechanical ventilation, researchers found a decrease in length of stay and costs, but these reductions were not statistically significant (Burns et al., 1998). This study was based on evaluating the use of pathways as a means of "outcome management." Although there was no significant effect demonstrated, the investigators speculated that all clinicians, even those caring for patients in the control groups, "may have learned from the outcomes-managed approach, thus biasing the study and diminishing any potential effect ... "(p. 56). Anecdotal evidence that supports the benefits of using pathways includes a demonstrated improvement in communications among physicians, nurses, other staff, family members, and clients (Mosher, Cronk, Kidd, McCormick, Stockton, & Sulla, 1992), improved teamwork and coordination of care delivered by all the different disciplines involved with orthopaedic elective surgery (Poole & Johnson, 1996), and as "powerful mechanisms to prevent malpractice litigation" (Forkner, 1996, p. 35) because of their clarity in describing crucial areas of malpractice vulnerability.

Care pathways are the standards of care for a given condition in a given setting; quality is measured by degree of conformance to the standards as defined in the CP. At the national level, the Agency for Health Care Policy and Research (AHCPR) has developed standards to be used to guide care for selected conditions. These standards are called protocols, but contain the same elements as the critical pathways described above, although protocols are often more general and not as useful for staff trying to plan care. The process used to develop standards, whether they are referred to as pathways, guidelines, or protocols, is similar groups of experts collaborate in the review of evidence to substantiate the critical elements of practice specific to the condition studied that will result in desired outcomes. Thus, CPs, protocols, and guidelines are data-based standards for practice. These standards can be a most effective tool in the hands of a professional such as the APN, who can use them to teach other staff or to guide the care provided by nonlicensed personnel in nursing homes and home care.

The idea of developing standards is arguably a good one (Kane, 1995). However, one of the major problems facing caregivers attempting to use these standards in a managed care system is that they are setting-specific. That is, they have been developed to guide the care in a given institution, and do not provide guidance for transition of care across settings. They include only short-term outcomes that are specific to discharge from that setting. Although these short-term outcomes may not stand in direct contradiction to long-term outcomes of care, there is no attention given to how they might support the long-term goals or serve as intermediate measures of progress toward long-term outcomes. There is a need to someone to interpret the CP to various caregivers in various settings and to use the standard encompassed to determine what modifications are necessary to meet the needs of the individual client. The person most qualified to do this interpretation is the APN. The APN has specialized knowledge about the client population for which the standard was written, and understands how to assess, plan, and evaluate what cares are necessary to produce the desired client outcome. It is the APN, after all, who has the picture of the whole client and all his or her needs over time. The goal of the client, whatever it may be, is at the heart of process—what needs to be done in order to achieve the outcome. The APN is in the best position to know this information and to use it in the interest of the client.

To illustrate the need for articulation among settings, let us return to the case of Mr. H. Few elderly clients with hip fracture return home directly from the hospital. Most are discharged to a nursing home or a rehabilitation facility. Those who do go home require the support of a home caregiver. Without an overall plan for continuous care that encompasses the whole episode and that guides specific aspects of care over time, each caregiver is left to devise his or her own plan. This plan may or may not fit with care plans from other settings, with the longer-term recovery plan, or with the client's unspoken plan for the future. Indeed, Mr. H was not involved in planning at all. It seems that no one has the whole picture in mind of the course that the client should follow in order to achieve the desired outcomes. Hence, Mr. H's experience has been one of care that has been discontinuous, fragmented, unnecessarily redundant at times, and generally ineffective for achieving long-term wellness outcomes. The team approach certainly has the advantage of bringing together professionals with expertise and experience with patients in the nursing home. However, it remains focused on the nursing home, and on Mr. H's progress there toward the outcome of discharge. How much better care would be for Mr H if an APN were coordinating his care according to a standard agreed upon by the team and applicable across settings.

A more recent development that seeks to address this concern about disjointed planning is the Extended Care Pathway (ECP). This tool has all the elements of a CP; however, it encompasses the whole continuum of care for a specific problem or condition. It describes the outcomes to be achieved, the specific interventions to be carried out and by whom, the time frame, and the key factors to be addressed in order to effect the desired outcomes over time and regardless of setting. An example of an ECP for hip fracture is included as Figure 6.1.

FIGURE 6.1 OUTCOMES-FOCUSED CARE MANAGEMENT (OuTCM) MODEL FOR CARE OF ELDERLY WITH HIP FRACTURES

Kathleen Krichbaum, RN, PhD

KEY FACTORS	EPISODE RECOVERY OUTCOMES			RECOVERY OUTCOMES WELLNESS
	ACUTE CARE MANAGEMENT (0-5 days)	INTERMEDIATE OUTCOMES SUBACUTE CARE MANAGEMENT (6-19 days)	MOBILITY CARE MANAGEMENT (20 4 5 days)	MANAGEMENT (46 180 days)

HEALTH STATUS
• Physical
  - walking capacity
  - muscle strength
  - pain
  - physiological
  - nutrition stability
 	
• Mental
 	
• Psychological/Social
 	
• Co-Morbidities/Medications
	HEALTH STATUS
	• Physiologically Stable
	• Fracture Repaired
	• Pain Managed
	• Muscle Strength Assessed
	• Ambulates in Room with Assistance
	• Nutrition Assessed
	
	• Alert, Oriented
	• Cognitive Level Assessed
	• Clinical Depression Assessed
	• Social history completed
	• Co-Morbidities Managed
	• Takes Medications as Pre-Fracture
		HEALTH STATUS
		• Physiologically Stable
		• States Pain Controlled
		• Demonstrates adequate muscle strength
		• Transfers Independently
		• Ambulates Self with Assistive Device
		• Adequate Nutrition
		• Alert, Oriented
		
		• Clinical Depression Managed as needed
		• Co-Morbidities Stable
		• Takes Medications as Pre-Fracture
			HEALTH STATUS
			• Demonstrates Adequate Muscle Strength
			• Ambulates as Desired
			• States Health as "good or very good"
			• Adequate Nutrition
			
			• Mental Status Stable
			
			• Depression Managed as needed
			• Co-Morbidities Managed Including Medications
				HEALTH STATUS
				□ Demonstrates Adequate Muscle Strength
				□ Ambulates Equal to Pre-Fracture
				□ Adequate Nutrition
				□ States Health as Equal to or Better than Pre-Fracture
				
				□ Mental Status as Pre-Fracture
				□ Depression Resolved
				
				□ Co-Morbidities Stable and Managed

LEVEL OF INDEPENDENCE • ADLs • IADLs	**LEVEL OF INDEPENDENCE** • Feeds, Grooms Self • Dresses Upper Self • Toilets with Assist	**LEVEL OF INDEPENDENCE** □ Independent in all ADLs □ IADL Management Assessed	**LEVEL OF INDEPENDENCE** • All ADLs as Pre-fracture • All IADLs as Pre-Fracture	**LEVEL OF INDEPENDENCE** □ All ADLs equal to Pre-Fracture □ All IADLs equal to Pre-Fracture
DISCHARGE ENVIRONMENT • Homesite • Presence of Caregiver	**ENVIRONMENT** • States desired discharge site • Identifies Caregiver	**ENVIRONMENT** • Discharge Environment Assessed	**ENVIRONMENT** • Safe Environment • Knows Resources Available	**ENVIRONMENT** □ Living at Home □ Decreased Risk for Falls
SELF MANAGEMENT ABILITY • Level of knowledge • Level of skill	**HEALTH MANAGEMENT** • Knowledge Assessed • Skills Assessed	**HEALTH MANAGEMENT** • States Wellness Goal • Demonstrates Knowledge of Co-Morbidity Management • States Plan for Care	**HEALTH MANAGEMENT** • Able to state plan of care • Demonstrates Skill in self-care • Demonstrates knowledge of condition • Care Manager Consults	**HEALTH MANAGEMENT** □ Satisfied □ Manages independently
• Care Manager Introduced	• Plan for Care Management Developed/Individualized with client	• Family Caregiver Evolved; Educated in Care Management		□ Care Manager withdraws

This ECP was developed by an interdisciplinary team in a large integrated care system. Disciplines represented included nursing, physical therapy, occupational therapy, social work, and medicine. The time frame for recovery is 6 months; the key factors to be addressed include the patient's comorbidities and total health profile (physical health, mental health, psychosocial health, nutrition), the level of independence, the environment in which recovery takes place (regardless of institution) and the education of the patient and all caregivers (self-management ability). Figure 6.1 actually represents the model used to develop the ECP; the actual pathway is much longer and even more detailed. It was designed to fit the type of documentation used in each setting where the patient might be transferred during the 6 months of recovery. This pathway was designed based on the current information available on hip fracture recovery and on the experiences of the professionals who developed the pathway with elderly patients who have fractured a hip. It is built on specific client recovery needs rather than on the needs of the setting. Thus, it transcends the setting and focuses on achievement of patient outcomes. The idea of having the client be at the center of the process of care and recovery is a nursing concept, one that is basic to the practice of the APN.

There has been interest nationally in the development and use of ECPs. The National Chronic Care Consortium has established guidelines for ECP development. However, to date no studies have been completed that validate the effectiveness of ECPs for improving either the long-term processes or outcomes of care.

The ECP described above was pilot-tested in 1997. The pilot demonstrated the relevance of the key factors identified for recovery. We also found that in order to acquaint staff with this very different approach to patient care planning in each of the care settings, extensive orientation was necessary (Krichbaum, 1997). Patient information that was fundamental to long-range planning still seemed to get lost in between agencies. In progress is a study funded by the National Institute for Nursing Research (K01-NR000094) that tests the effectiveness of the ECP in the hands of a Gerontologic Advanced Practice Nurse to improve outcomes for patients over the age of 65 with hip fracture.

A tool is only as good as the person who uses it. In the hands of APNs, CPs, and ECPs hold promise for the improvement of care in terms of both efficiency and effectiveness for achieving outcomes. However, further definition of the scope of the role of the APN within the health care delivery system is necessary to achieve the desired client outcomes.

CASE MANAGEMENT: THE TECHNIQUE OF CHOICE IN MANAGED CARE

The term "case management," describes an approach used in today's health care environment for controlling the costs while ensuring quality. While the term "managed care" refers to the systems of administration used to coordinate services and care providers, case management refers to the service itself, carried out by professionally educated individuals who provide and/or coordinate health and social services (Eggert, Bowlyow, & Nichol, 1991). It encompasses a set of logical steps and a process of interaction within a service network that assures that patients receive needed services in a supportive, efficient, and effective manner. These "logical steps" have been described in various ways, but generally include functions such as case-finding, assessment of patient needs, care planning, implementation, monitoring, and evaluation. Although there exist multiple definitions of case management, R. A. Kane, Urv-Wong, & King (1990) state that the "litmus test" for case management for persons with long-term care needs consists of the following criteria: (1) a population focus, (2) continuity of attention, (3) coordination of services, (4) comprehensive, periodic assessments to determine progress over time, and (5) construction of information systems that permit better allocation of services. If one considers the practice of APNs, it is easy to match that practice to these criteria; the scope of the role of the APN goes beyond these functions, however.

As a means of service coordination, case management has been in existence for over one hundred years. In 1863, the state of Massachusetts attempted to institute a system to coordinate public human services and conserve public funds used to care for the poor and sick. From these beginnings, the use of social workers to manage cases probably arose. Within the nursing profession, case management was introduced by Lillian Wald in 1895 to provide services at home for individual patients referred by their doctors. In this first public health model, the nurse coordinated care between the physician and family and arranged for admission to the hospital, if necessary. Nurses in Wald's Henry Street settlement also worked to provide the poor with necessities of life they were unable to afford (Kalisch & Kalisch, 1986). In the 1940s, the notion of "continuum of care" was introduced to describe the extended, outpatient services needed by psychiatric patients discharged into the community. There were no services available, however, until 1962, when the President's Commission on Mental Retardation recommended a program coordinator to facilitate the patient's access to services, and to serve as the link between the hospital and the patient in the community. Since that time, the role of psychiatric case manager has evolved to include reducing the use of state mental hospitals, improving continuity of care, and enhancing the patient and family's quality of life outside the institution (Franklin, Solovitz, Mason, Clemons, & Miller, 1987).

In 1971, the Allied Services Act proposed to integrate health, education, and welfare programs for elderly patients in need of long-term care. Demonstration projects spawned by this act illustrated the success of case managers in providing ways to accomplish that integration. With the advent of diagnostic-related groups (DRGs) for reimbursement of hospital care in 1983, the length of stay for patients has steadily decreased. Patients are discharged early and in a sicker state, necessitating transfer to subacute facilities, transitional care facilities, or to home with a need for services. Hospitals have developed a system of discharge planning that often includes the use of a nurse or social worker to act as a "case manager" to coordinate services necessary to support patients outside of acute care. Although the term "case manager" exists, its meaning varies depending on the organization or system in which it is used. Often, it is restricted to one agency, and does not provide the desired link between agencies or between hospital and home.

Although case management as a technique within managed care or as a philosophy of service delivery has grown in popularity, much of the literature is anecdotal. Research about its effectiveness in relation to client outcomes is scant. Studies to date have examined case management in terms of three types of system variables: (1) variables addressing the structures supporting care delivery, (2) process variables that define care interventions, and (3) outcome variables that can be observed as a result of patients experiencing managed care. No comprehensive study of all three types of variables affecting case management has yet been completed.

In the studies of structural variables, case management was described as conducted by a variety of departments using teams of care providers consisting of a physician, nurse, and social worker. Case management procedures were developed within hospitals to oversee the patient's stay from preadmission through discharge planning (Eggert et al., 1991). In a review of the literature, Marschke and Nolan (1993) reviewed research on case management as a process used to manage care. Generally, the need for services provided to patients following discharge from an acute care institution decreased over time when these patients were followed by case managers. Results were mixed, however, in relation to types of services provided and cost-effectiveness of case management (Franklin et al., 1987; Hurley, Paul, & Freund, 1989; Polinsky, Fred, & Ganz, 1991). These studies were methodologically flawed in that they lacked control groups and/or similar definitions of case management.

Studies of outcomes resulting from the use of case management are increasing. In one, the use of resources with patients needing caesarean section were compared between two groups. The group with case management required more resources, but resulted in cost savings due to decreased length of stay (Cohen, 1991). In another study, birth outcomes of Medicaid recipients receiving managed care were compared to those who did not receive it. Investigators found that managed care had no effect on prenatal care received or on birth weight outcomes (Krieger, Connell, & LoGerfo, 1992). The exact nature of the managed care system used was not clear, however, making it difficult to generalize the findings.

The classic study in nursing that demonstrated the effectiveness of professional nurse case managers (PNCMs) was conducted at Carondelet St. Mary's Hospital and Health Center in Tucson, Arizona (Etheridge & Lamb, 1989). Nurses within this integrated system of care comprised the Nursing Network that included acute care inpatient, extended care/long-term care, home care, hospice, and ambulatory care services. Patient movement among these services was coordinated by the PNCM. The PNCM assessed patient and family, developed the care plan, delegated care to associates as appropriate, activated interventions, collaborated with the multidisciplinary team, and evaluated outcomes. Reduction in length of stay and costs was accomplished in case-managed patients, despite the fact that PNCM-managed patients had a higher average acuity that non-case managed patients. Further, patients with chronic illnesses managed by PNCMs had lower costs in terms of hospitalization, due to the PNCM's ability to provide early access to acute care when necessary (the coordinator role).

More recent literature includes descriptions of many new models of case management. Tartre-Lemire (1996) describes a model based on a preclinical entry point for case managers in which consumers are involved as they are enrolled into a managed care plan. Using social cognitive theory, the case manager assists the patient's self-efficacy behaviors, such as goal-setting and resource utilization, before problems arise. Strumpf (1994) describes several successful programs in which nurse case managers have worked with elderly clients to produce better long-term care outcomes.

It is apparent from these studies that more investigation of case management for its impact on outcomes is needed. Most effort has gone into elaborating the process, a necessary yet not sufficient step. As organizations strive for effectiveness and efficiency in case management, it seems that the best models will emerge and can be applied to a variety of settings. Before that occurs, however, there needs to be a universal definition of case management. Comparisons can then be made about which models work best and who provides the most effective service. If our patient with a hip fracture, Mr. H., had had an APN case manager who knew him and his family, how would his course of care been affected? How would his experience have been different? Despite the lack of empirical evidence to support its effectiveness, most would agree that case management makes sense as a technique that has potential to reduce problems that occur due to lack of continuity.

WHO BEST TO MANAGE CARE ACROSS THE CONTINUUM?

Because of the lack of agreement about what constitutes effective case management, there exists much debate about who should best assume the role. Wolfe (1993) makes the point that as long as there is money to be made, there will be competition for the job of case manager.

In an essay about nursing case management, Newman, Lamb, & Michaels (1991) discuss case management as the perfect vehicle for practicing professional nursing. They say that case management, "exemplifies the essence of nursing that was always there but was overshadowed at times by the response to external demands," (p. 405). They cite the work done at Carondelet, where nurses work with patients within the system of care delivery that crosses settings (Etheridge & Lamb, 1989). The patient is a partner; the nurse has the authority to make care decisions and to obtain necessary services based on his or her judgement about what is needed. This non-hierarchical, collegial model of practice provides a network within which collaboration can occur around issues that affect patients' recovery.

Although nurses in the Carondelet model were not all APNs, the matching of professional nursing and case management is long overdue. Nurses have always performed the functions of case management, restricted in their ability to make care decisions only by the agency that employed them. Nursing theory is based on the relationship between the nurse and patient, who is, and should be, the focus of the case management activity. Furthermore, nurses have always used care plans—tools that map out the necessary interventions and outcomes—to assess, plan, intervene, and evaluate the process used to produce the desired outcomes in patients. APNs have the added benefit of specialized knowledge and expertise with the specific client population that greatly enhances their understanding of the client's needs and of the scope of possibilites for interventions to achieve desired outcomes.

Returning to our discussion of Mr. H., let us assume that he had an APN care manager at the time of his fracture, someone who could assess him regularly based on comparisons to a baseline assessment done at the time of his admission to his managed care provider. This APN could work with Mr. H., set mutual goals based on knowledge of him and his wife and family, and would recognize his depression as variance from his norm. The APN would help the family decide about the best place for rehabilitation based on knowing the resources available and costs. The APN would attend all team care planning meetings, leading the discussion as expert in Mr. H.'s case. The therapies Mr. H. was receiving would be part of a comprehensive plan described on the Extended Care Pathway, and interpreted by the APN, who would work with the therapists to monitor and evaluate progress. The APN would order antibiotics, if necessary, and perhaps could have avoided the incidence of iatrogenic UTI in the first place. The family would know what to expect, and Mr. H. would know what it meant to fracture his hip and what to do to recover. How much better off Mr. H. would be with someone who had knowledge of the whole continuum of care to work with him, someone who knows him and his family, someone who he could trust to be with him for the whole recovery period. APN care managers with responsibility and authority for following clients through the system, using standards decided upon by multidisciplinary teams, could revolutionize the system. More importantly, they could revolutionize the way that clients experience the system—as a system of health care, rather than as episodes of illness care in which they are "treated and released".

The recent expansion of the role of APNs in primary care opens the door to nurses being able to take on greater responsibility and to demonstrate increasing accountability for outcomes. Third-party reimbursement for services places nurses squarely at the cutting edge of revolutionizing health care. Nurses can begin to control resources for meeting their patients' needs and can leverage that control to provide for effectiveness and efficiency in the delivery of care. As nurses, we must learn to use the tools, like care pathways, and the techniques, like case management, to help our patients navigate the health care system. We must learn to manage care ourselves, as we have demonstrated we can do, rather than being managed by the system.

REFERENCES

Aiken, L. (1990). *Educational innovations in gerontology: Teaching nursing homes and gerontological nurse practitioners.* Washington, DC.: Association for Gerontology in Higher Education.

Aiken, L. H., Lake, E. T., Semaan, S., Lehman, H. P., O'Hare, P. A., Cole, C. S., Dunbar, D., & Frank, I. (1993). Nurse Practitioner managed care for persons with HIV infection. *Journal of Nursing Scholarship, 25*(3), 172–177.

Brooten, D., Brown, L., Hazarck-Munro, B., York, R., Cohen, S., Roncoli, U., & Hollingsworth, A. (1988). Early discharge and specialist transitional care. *Image, 20*(2), 64–68.

Brooten, D., Kumar, S., Brown, L., Butts, P., Finkler, S., Bakewell-Sachs, S., & Gibbons, A. (1986). A randomized clinical trial of early hospital discharge and follow-up of very low birthweight infants. *New England Journal of Medicine, 35,* 934–939.

Brooten, D., & Naylor, M. (1994). Nurses' effect on changing patient outcomes. *Image, 27*(2), 95–99.

Burgess, A., Learner, D., D'Agostino, R., Vokonas, P., Hartman, C., & Gaccione, P. (1987). A randomized clinical trial of cardiac rehabilitation. *Social Science and Medicine, 24,* 359–370.

Burl, J. B., Bonner, A., Rao, M. & Kahn, A. M. (1998). Geriatric Nurse Practitioner in long-term care: Demonstration of effectiveness in managed care. *Journal of the American Geriatrics Society, 46*(4), 506–510.

Burns, S. M., Marshall, M., Burns, J. E., Ryan, B., Wilmoth, D., Carpenter, R., Aloi, A., Wood, M., & Truwit, J. D. (1998). Design, testing, and results of an outcomes-managed approach to patients requiring prolonged mechanical ventilation. *American Journal of Critical Care, 7*(1), 45–57.

Coffey, R., Richards, J., Remmert, C., LeRoy, S., Schoville, R., & Boldwin, P. (1992). *Quality Management in Health Care, 1*(1), 45–54.

Cohen, E. L. (1991). Nursing case management: Does it pay? *Journal of Nursing Administration, 21*(4), 20–25.

Deming, W. E. (1989). *Out of the crisis.* Cambridge, MA: Massachusetts Institute of Technology, Center for Advanced Engineering Studies.

Eggert, G. M., Bowlyow, J., & Nichol, C. W. (1991). Case management: A randomized controlled study comparing a neighborhood team and a centralized individual model. *Health Services Research, 26,* 471–507.

Etheredge, M. L. S. (Ed.). (1989). *Collaborative care: Nursing case management.* Chicago, IL: American Hospital Publishing.

Ethridge, P., & Lamb, G. S. (1989). Professional nursing case management improves quality, access and costs. *Nursing Management, 20*(3), 30–35.

Forkner, D. J. (1996). Clinical pathways: Benefits and liabilities. *Nursing Management, 27*(11), 35–38.

Franklin, J., Solovitz, B., Mason, M., Clemons, J. R., & Miller, G. E. (1987). An evaluation of case management. *American Journal of Public Health, 77,* 674–678.

Gartner, M. B., & Twardon, C. A. (1995). Care guidelines: Journey through the managed care maze. *JWOCN, 22*(3), 118–121.

Hurley, R., Paul, J. E., & Freund, D. (1989). Going into gatekeeping: An empirical assessment. *Quality Review Bulletin, 15,* 306–314.

Inouye, S., Acampora, D., Miller, R., Fulmer, T., Hurst, L., & Cooney, L. (1993). The Yale Geriatric Care Program: A model of care to prevent functional decline in hospitalized elderly patients. *Journal of the American Geriatrics Society, 41*(12), 1345–1352.

Kalisch, P., & Kalisch, B. (1986). *The advance of American nursing* (2nd ed.). New York: Little, Brown.

Kane, R., Garrard, J., Buchanan, J., Rosenfeld, A., Skay, C., & McDermott, S. (1991). Improving care in nursing homes. *Journal of American Geriatrics Society, 39*(4), 359–367.

Kane, R. A., Kane, R. L., Arnold, S., Garrard, J., McDermott, S., & Kepferle, L. (1988). Geriatric nurse practitioners as nursing home employees: Implementing the role. *The Gerontologist, 28*(4) 469–477.

Kane, R. A., Urv-Wong, K., & King, C. (Eds.) (1990). *Case management: What is it anyway?* Minneapolis, MN: University of Minnesota Long-Term Care Decisions Resource Center.

Kane, R. L. (1995). Creating practice guidelines: The dangers of over-reliance on expert judgement. *Journal of Law, Medicine & Ethics, 23,* 62–64.

Kane, R. L., Garrard, J., Arnold, S., Kane, R. A., & McDermott, S. (1989). Assessing the effectiveness of geriatric nurse practioners. In M. D. Mezey, J. E. Lynaugh, & M. M. Cartier (Eds.), *Nursing homes and nursing care: Lessons from the teaching nursing homes* (pp. 203–217). New York: Springer Publishing Company.

Koch, M. O., & Smith, J. A., Jr. (1996). Influence of patient age and co-morbidity on outcome of a collaborative care pathway after radical prostatectomy and cystoprostatectomy. *Journal of Urology, 155,* 1681–1684.

Krichbaum, K. (1997). *The extended care pathway for elders with hip fracture: A pilot study.* Unpublished manuscript.

Krieger, J. W., Connell, F. A., & Logerfo, J. P. (1992). Medicaid prenatal care: A comparison of use and outcomes in fee-for-service and managed care. *American Journal of Public Health, 82*(2), 185–190.

Mabrey, J. D., Toohey, J. S., Armstrong, D. A., Lavery, L., & Wammack, L. A.

(1997). Clinical pathway management of total knee arthroplasty. *Clinical Orthopaedics and Related Research, 345,* 125–133.

Marschke, P., & Nolan, M. (1993). Research related to case management. *Nursing Administration Quarterly, 17*(3), 16–21.

McCorkle, R. (1989). The complications of early discharge from hospitals. *Proceedings of the 5ᵗʰ National Conference: Human Values & Cancer.* New York: American Cancer Society.

Mezey, M., & Lynaugh, J. (1989). The teaching nurse home program: Outcomes of care. *Nursing Clinics of North America, 24*(3), 769–780.

Mosher, C., Cronk, P., Kidd, A., McCormick, P., Stockton, S., & Sulla, C. (1992). Upgrading practice with critical pathways. *American Journal of Nursing, 92,* 41–44.

Naylor, M. (1990). Comprehensive discharge planning for hospitalized elderly: A pilot study. *Nursing Research, 39*(3), 156–161.

Naylor, M., & Brooten, D. (1993). The roles and functions of clinical nurse specialists. *Image, 25*(1), 73–78.

Naylor, M., Brooten, D., Jones, R. Lavizzo-Mouvey, R., Mezey, M., & Pauly, M. (1994). Comprehensive discharge planning for hospitalized elderly: A randomized clinical trial. *Annals of Internal Medicine, 120*(12), 999–1006.

Neidlinger, S., Scroggins, K., & Kennedy, L. (1987). Cost evaluation of discharge planning for hospitalized elderly. *Nursing Economics, 5*(5), 225–230.

Newman, M., Lamb, G. S. & Michaels, C. (1991). Nurse case management: The coming together of theory and practice. *Nursing and Health Care, 12*(8), 404–408.

Noedel, N., Osterloh, J., Brannan, J., Haselhorst, M., Ramage, L., & Lambrechts, D. (1996). Critical pathways as an effective tool to reduce cardiac transplantation rehospitalization and charges. *Journal of Transplant Coordination, 6*(1), 14–19.

Office of Technology Assessment. (1986). *Nursing practitioners, physician assistants, and certified nurse midwives: A policy analysis* (Health Technology Care Study 37, OTA-HCS-37). Washington, DC: U.S. Government Printing Office.

Pew Health Professions Commission. (1995). *Executive summary: A new world for health care.* San Francisco, CA: UCSF Center for the Health Professions.

Polinsky, M. L., Fred, C., & Ganz, P. (1991). Quantitative and qualitative assessment of a case management program for cancer patients. *Health and Social Work, 16,* 176–183.

Poole, P., & Johnson, S. (1996). Integrated care pathways: An orthopaedic experience. *Physiotherapy, 82*(1), 28–30.

Riley, S. A. (1994). Clinical pathways: A basic tool for subacute care. *Nursing Homes, July/August,* 35–36.

Ryden, M., Snyder, M., Krichbaum, K., Mueller, C., Gross, C., & Savik, K.

(1998). *Value-added outcomes: The use of Advanced Practice Nurses in long-term care facilities.* Unpublished manuscript.

Safriet, B. (1992). Health care dollars and regulatory sense: The role of advance practice nursing. *Yale Journal on Regulation, 9*(2), 417–487.

Schaldach, D. E. (1997). Measuring quality and cost of care: Evaluation of an amputation clinical pathway. *Journal of Vascular Nursing, 15*(1), 13–20.

Strumpf, N. E. (1994). Innovative gerontological practices as models for health care delivery. *Nursing & Health Care, 15*(10), 522–527.

Tartre-Lemire, E. (1996). Community-based health reform: A case management model for consumer self-determination. *Journal of Care Management, 2*(3), 9–26.

Wolfe, G. (1993). Cooperation or competition? *Caring magazine, 12*(10), 52–60.

Zander, K. (1988). Nursing case management: Strategic management of cost and quality outcomes. *Journal of Nursing Administration, 8,* 2–30.

Chapter 7

THE APN AS EDUCATOR

Rita Kisting Sparks, RN, PhD

The Pew Health Professions Commission, in its *Agenda for Action* (1991), identified societal changes which will affect the preparation of health care professionals for the year 2005. To contain health care costs, they projected a more coordinated, managed care system with greater focus on health of the total population rather than the individual; a mix of health care providers; and mechanisms to continually and systematically measure outcomes to assess quality and hold practitioners accountable. Increased diversity and aging in the population necessitate a refocusing on chronic health problems, especially on education to help persons prevent or live with their health problems. The emphasis on "cure" will shift to "care". Expansion of knowledge in science and technology, which have brought the public greater diagnostic and therapeutic capabilities, will require a balancing of the depersonalization driven by technology with a humanistic focus on consumer choice and quality of life. The public is demanding a system that integrates technology with humanism. Nurses in advanced practice roles have a responsibility to be leaders in this movement.

Consumer empowerment must occur to respond to the consumer demand for a part in decisions regarding their health, therefore increasing the emphasis on health promotion. Health care providers have a responsibility to provide information to consumers on which consumers can base their decisions. Cost, convenience, and quality will be a part of these decisions.

The Pew Commission (1991) identified a rising tension between the core values of the rights of the individual and importance of the common good. Nurses in advanced practice will need to be prepared to participate fully in decisions which affect use of limited resources, access to care, or quality versus extension of life. Knowledge transmission is essential in this process.

STRATEGIES FOR EDUCATORS

In the era of self-care and responsibility for ones own health, the need for patient/client education is greater than ever before. Simsek and Heydinger (1992), in their presentation on the managed populism present in higher education in the 1990s, identified five key strategies for educators. These strategies are useful for nurses in advanced practice, particularly when examining their educator function.

Focus on the Customer

Advanced practice nurses (APNs) have many customers. However, nurses usually focus on one primary customer at a time. As experts, nurses in advanced practice must assume responsibility not only for client and family education, but for educating colleagues, novice nurses, nursing students, and members of the community as well. APNs must stay in close touch with the customers to determine their needs and select the strategies to best meet those needs.

Be Specific and Demanding About Quality

Quality is defined as "meeting or exceeding the expectations of those who are served" (Simsek & Heydinger, 1992, p. 35). Assessment of needs is the first step in assuring quality; evaluation of outcomes must be done to determine effectiveness of the teaching and other services designed to meet these needs.

Build From Collaboration

As in the field of higher education, collaboration in the health care arena is essential. The nurse in advanced practice needs to work with other health care providers to assure the timely delivery of education to meet the needs of clients.

Utilize Technology to its Fullest

Technology can be a means of delivering education to clients efficiently. This presumes that the assessment of need has been done, that a prepared teaching plan is available to meet that need, and that the client has access to the technology. With greater access to computers, teaching may be done via the Internet. Consumers can search the world wide web for information about their health problems. Practitioners can search for solutions to problems via the web, listserve, or groupware. Unfortunately some of the information accessed may be inaccurate. Just as printed teaching materials need to be evaluated for quality, so too must Web-based education be evaluated. Assessment of need, interpretations, clarification, and determination of understanding continue to be necessary. Teaching via distance learning methods is becoming more feasible as states establish statewide transmission networks. Many health care institutions have purchased equipment to gain access to national education programs. However, easy access is not always possible for learners, especially in rural communities. A key ingredient in any teaching/learning endeavor, however, is the determination of whether the selected teaching strategies have been effective and learning has resulted. In many instances, optimal learning requires personal contact with the teacher who, in this instance, is the nurse.

Recognize the Inherent Power of Accountability Measures

Nurses in advanced practice are, first and foremost, accountable to their clients. They are also accountable to their employer and the profession of nursing. Data collected to demonstrate accountability of nurses in advanced practice roles can be used to justify their effective and efficient use in the health care arena.

Historically, nurses in advanced practice roles have viewed education as one of their primary roles, whether they function as a clinical nurse specialist, nurse practitioner, certified registered nurse anesthestist, or certified nurse midwife. The role of the clinical nurse specialist has a strong component of team-building and team support. The CNS's effectiveness has been frequently measured by how effective the team was in reaching mutual goals. It is not surprising, then, that many CNSs have placed a high value on education and spent a large segment of their time performing the educator role (Hart, Lekander, Bartels, & Tebbitt, 1987; Taristano, Brophy, & Snyder, 1986). Robichaud and Hamric (1986) found CNSs spent 27% of their time on staff, student, and community education. Patient education was considered a part of direct patient care, to which CNSs attributed 40% of their time.

Nurse practitioners identified the teaching-coaching function as one of the major areas of their practice (Brykczynski, 1989). In a comparative study, Elder and Bullough (1990) found a high proportion of both nurse practitioners and clinical nurse specialists reported they were involved with teaching patients (96%), families (80%), counseling (77%), and psychosocial assessment (69%). The researchers found no significant difference between the two groups on any of these functions.

ADVANCED PRACTICE NURSES AS ADULT LEARNERS/ TEACHERS

The profession of nursing, through the American Nurses' Association (ANA), has declared that preparation of advanced practice nurses be at the graduate level, with minimal qualifications being a master''s degree and national professional certification. When the profession moved to this requirement, those ANA certified nurses without graduate preparation were grandpersoned as certified specialists (CS). Therefore, there are nurses in advance practice roles who do not have a master's degree.

An expectation of all professional nurses, including those in advanced practice, is continued, lifelong learning. Nurses in advanced practice recognize the need for gaining the necessary skills and knowledge as well as keeping up to date on changes in health care and nursing practice. To assure that certified nurses are maintaining currency through continuing education, the American Nurses' Credentialing Center and other certifying agencies require a specific number of hours of continuing education in specified areas for the nurse to be recertified.

Advanced practice nurses have not only a commitment to their own continued learning but also assume responsibility for providing continuing education for other nurses. Therefore, assumptions about adult learning are relevant for advanced practice nurses not only from the perspective of the learner, but also of the teacher. These assumptions are helpful in all phases of the teaching-learning process, from assessment and planning to implementation and evaluation. They are relevant in teaching all persons, regardless of age. Knowles and Associates (1984), in their andragogical model of learning, identified the assumptions as:

1. *The learner is self-directing:* Learners are responsible for their own lives, including learning. They need to have a sense of control over what is learned and how.
2. *Experience is a rich resource for learning:* Adult learners have a wealth of life experiences on which to build new learning. Educators must learn with the learner how to use these experiences in the teaching-learning situation.
3. *Readiness to learn occurs with a perceived need to know or do something* Learning is related to the problems or the role expectations with which the person is dealing.
4. *Orientation to learning is problem-centered or task-centered:* Learning experiences must be relevant to the learner's current life tasks or problems; content must be applicable to his/her immediate situation.
5. *Internal motivation is more potent than external motivators:* The teacher takes into consideration the learner's values, expectations, motivations, and self-esteem. Determining how the content relates to the learner's quality of life, self-confidence, or movement toward self-actualization is needed.

The andragogical model focuses on process design. A dual role is assigned to the facilitator/teacher. The first and primary role is that of designer and manager of processes which will facilitate learning of the content by the learners. Secondarily, the educator assumes the role of content resource. The model assumes there are many resources other than the teacher, including peers, colleagues, community resources, and media. The teacher makes available such resources as they think are relevant for the learning experience. The androgogical model includes seven basic process design elements which are presented in Table 7.1.

Care is directed toward the physical environment as well as the psy-

TABLE 7.1   Elements of Androgogical Process Design

Climate-setting
Involve learners in mutual planning
Involve learners in diagnosing own learning needs
Involve learners in formulating learning objectives
Involve learners in designing learning plans
Help learners carry out their learning plans
Involve learners in evaluating their learning

Note: Adapted from "Andragogy in Action" (pp. 14–18), by M. S. Knowles, 1984, San Francisco: Jossey-Bass.

chological environment. The physical environment is as user-friendly as the content and learning experiences allow. It is important to arrange the room to allow eye contact between the presenter and participants and to the extent possible, between participants. Bright rooms are desired, but lighting needs to be adjusted to allow visualization of media. The setting should allow learners to focus on the educational experience without distractions from noise or other persons.

To ensure a psychological climate which is conducive to learning, a climate of mutual respect is necessary. Feeling respected comes with acknowledgement of one's worth; learners' experiences are treated as important. A climate of collaborativeness is facilitated by allowing learners to share their thoughts and experiences; colleagues learn much from each other. A climate of mutual trust is encouraged by placing decisions in the learners' hands. A climate of supportiveness can be promoted by interactions of the teacher/facilitator with the learners or the structuring of activities which allow fellow learners to support each other. Allowing learners to share what they do and do not know, their accomplishments and their fears, helps build a climate of openness and authenticity. Education and learning needs to be fun, thus promoting a climate of pleasure.

Knowles et al. (1984) sum up their recommendations for climate-building by promoting a climate of humanness. This includes making sure the learners are comfortable, feel taken care of, and are cared about. The physical environment can be comfortable and the psychological climate can be caring, accepting, and social. Climate-setting becomes more of a challenge when the teaching/learning process occurs via distance education technologies. Contact may be via interactive television, compressed video, or a myriad of other routes. Though design of classrooms may help establish a climate of connectedness between partcipants, there may be many miles between teacher/learner and learner/learner.

Asynchronous learning via computers allows learners to establish their own comfort climate. They can access the learning space at their own time and place. Connections with other learners is via the words on the computer screen.

Learners need to feel as though they have some control over what is being taught, either via verbal or written surveys, or through assessments done at the beginning of the presentation or learning experience. Learners are given opportunities to have specific topics put on the agenda.

Involving participants in diagnosing their own needs for learning can be done formally or informally. Occasionally, learners need to learn what the institution, society, or health care professionals dictate. Providing the rationale for the needed content may help make the content more relevant to the learners.

Learning contracts are one way to involve learners in formulating their learning objectives. Contracts help learners identify what they need to learn. Learners describe the behaviors which will indicate if this knowledge has been obtained. Involving learners in designing learning plans assists the learner in identifying resources or strategies to accomplish the objective.

The nurse teacher may be needed to facilitate the learning either by presenting content, serving as or providing a resource, or structuring activities to help learners incorporate content into their existing cognitive field. It is often helpful to use multiple forms of teaching; for example, providing written pamphlets to the diabetic client as well as verbally discussing the disease and treatment. Demonstrating injections and having injection equipment available for learners to use during the teaching may also be helpful. With increased numbers of clients gaining health education from the Internet, it is essential that nurse providers clarify clients' understanding of the information.

The final component of the androgogical model is helping learners decide how they will validate that the objectives for learning were achieved. Finding measurable, yet meaningful, ways to demonstrate learning is sometimes challenging (Knowles et al., 1984).

There are many excellent reference sources on principles of learning and teaching strategies to which the nurse may wish to refer when planning a formal teaching presentation, either for an individual client, a family or a classroom presentation for students, health professionals, or the public (Caffarella, 1994; Farquharson, 1995; Kelly, 1992; Narrow, 1979; Rankin & Stallings, 1990; Rorden, 1987; Van Hoozer et al., 1987; Whitman, Graham, Gleit, & Boyd, 1992). A few guiding principles are included in Table 7.2 which are applicable to teaching on a one-to-one basis with a client, a family, or a group of nurses.

TABLE 7.2   Principles of Teaching

Proceed from the simple to the complex.
Build on what is known to learn the unknown.
Use terminology that is familiar to the learner.
Set short-term and long-term goals.
Plan a sequence of incremental learning activities.
Application of content enhances learning.
Learner objectives direct content and learning experiences.
Use positive reinforcement.
Evaluate outcomes of learning process.

ASSESSMENT OF NEED

Nurses in advanced practice have multiple audiences who will benefit from their expertise. Teaching of patients and families may be done as a part of direct patient care on an informal basis, rather than following a formal teaching plan. Teaching as a nursing intervention has the same need for assessment, planning, and evaluation as other types of interventions. Teaching community groups, nursing students or groups of colleagues in nursing and other health professions may be done more formally via lecture or discussion live or via distance education. Both types of teaching require consideration of the same processes of assessment, planning, intervention/teaching, and evaluation. Each of these processes will be discussed below, with consideration of both informal and formal teaching.

Whether teaching a client or a group of novice nurses, the first step in the teaching/learning process is assessment of the learner. Knowles (1970) defined a learning need as the "gap between the learner's present level of competence and a higher level of performance which is defined by the learner, the organization, or society" (p. 85). The APN assesses the learner's level of competence and the level at which the learner desires to operate, as well as what external forces, such as a professional nursing organization or the institution, define as the optimal level of achievement.

Learning needs assessment consists of investigation, validation, and communication (Puetz, 1992). The APN, as educator, searches for learning needs to be met so the nursing staff can reach a standard of care or the client can achieve self-care. Although it is important to include the learner in the identification of needs, the teacher often needs to provide some guidance. The needs assessment data are used as a baseline for evaluation activities. Once a need has been identified, validation is necessary to determine whether it is a result of lack of education or whether other factors prevent the nurse or client from performing as expected. This level of exploration may reveal organizational policies which inhibit the nurses performance, or a lack of resources for the client to act on prior education. Communicating the purpose as well as the results of the needs assessment is important so that persons involved know why they are being asked questions and why selected topics are being taught.

Needs assessments can be done in formal, semiformal, or informal ways. Formal methods include written assessments and interviews. A written pretest might be administered to a group of novice nurses to determine what data needs to be presented in a review class. An interview guide may be used to determine the learning needs of a diabetic client. Semiformal assessments include observations of performance or asking a group of nurses for input in a random fashion. Informal methods include follow-up of "we need . . ." statements or follow-up on client questions or concerns. Needs assessments must be adapted to the developmental level of the learner.

Initial assessment of the client learner includes data about the learners:

Ability to learn: This is not always easy to assess, as anxiety related to the situation may affect a person's ability to grasp what is said or written. However, the vocabulary the client uses may give the nurse an indication about the level of instruction which may be effective. Information sent via the Internet needs to be at a reading level for the lay population, if this is the intended audience.

Physical condition: Sensory impairments may interfere with the teaching/learning process. Fatigue or pain may affect a person's ability to concentrate.

Psychological readiness to learn: Timing or capturing the patient's readiness to learn has been identified as a key competency of nurse practitioners (Brykczynski, 1989). Readiness is determined by both verbal and nonverbal cues. Using the Internet to obtain information when the learner needs it can be very helpful.

Medical diagnoses/prognosis/treatment regimen: These factors not only provide cues about the content to be taught, but also allow the nurse to anticipate what questions clients might ask.

Nursing diagnoses: These should provide direction for the teaching to be done and the method of teaching which might be most effective.

Attitude/motivation: The way the clients view health or health problems will affect their perceived need to know. Motivating a client to change was identified by Brykczynski (1989) as a key competency of nurse practitioners.

Lifestyle: An important part of helping persons with chronic illnesses live with their condition is to help them integrate the implications of their illness and recovery into their lifestyle or adapt that lifestyle to meet their changed health care status and abilities. Teaching clients self-care was another key nurse practitioner competency identified by Brykczynski (1989).

Understanding of his/her illness: The client may view the illness differently than do health care professionals. Determining what meaning the condition has for the client may give the nurse guidance regarding teaching priorities. Information about almost any disease entity can be found on the Internet. As the accuracy of such information may be suspect, the nurse needs to explore with the client what information they have and clarify misunderstandings on correct misinformation. To address the concern about quality of consumer health resources, Medical Matrix (*www.medmatrix.org*) offers an "Internet Consumer Health Resources list," and Medline Plus, which is a new consumer health outreach effort of the National Library of Medicine (*www.nlm.nih.gov*).

As with other aspects of the nursing process, the outcome of the assessment of learning needs is the establishment of goals. However, it is important to validate assessment data and conclusions with the client, so that appropriate goals are set. If the data collected indicate several learning needs, the APN must establish priorities with the client. Priorities might be established based on hierarchy of needs, such as that of Maslow (1970) which indicates that survival needs are attended to before those related to safety and security, love, affection and belongingness, self-esteem and self-actualization. Priorities might also be based on the learner's need and the availability of the educator's time. An immediate or urgent need would be taken care of before a long-range need, a specific need before a more general need, and a survival need before a general well-being need (Whitman et al., 1992). At times, the educator may have the learners rank the importance of their own needs. At other times the nurse or the organization may need to establish priorities and goals based on client safety or organizational mission.

PLANNING PROCESS

Once goals of the teaching/learning process have been established, more specific learner objectives should be agreed upon. Whether or not objectives are formally written, a measurable endpoint to the teaching is established so both nurse and client know whether learning was achieved. Objectives should be clear, concise, and have the potential for attainment.

Three domains of learning objectives have been identified: cognitive, affective and psychomotor (Bloom, 1956). The cognitive domain is concerned with knowledge and information. The affective domain includes interests, values, or attitudes. Learning motor skills are included in the psychomotor domain. Table 7.3 gives examples of objectives for each domain.

This classification of objectives helps the educator plan appropriate, objective-specific teaching/learning strategies. Knowledge deficits can be managed by a variety of teaching strategies, including lectures, discussions, case studies, or independent study with videotapes, books, pamphlets or Web-based instruction. Psychomotor skill development requires small group or one-to-one teaching so that the skill can be taught and return demonstrations observed. The affective domain is the most challenging to teach and evaluate. Discussions, simulations, role-playing, or other interactive activities are helpful in bringing about attitudinal changes. The APN may be the educator for such programs or utilize others, such as psychologists, who have the knowledge or expertise required. It may be useful to refer to Bloom's (1956) taxonomy of educational objectives to identify desired levels of functioning in the three domains, proceeding from basic to higher levels of learning.

After objectives have been determined, the nurse plans what, how, when and where the teaching of the client will occur. The teaching may

TABLE 7.3   Examples of Learning Objectives for Each Domain

Domain of Learning	Learning Objectives
Cognitive	The patient will list three side effects of Dilantin.
Affective	The nurse participant joins the local district nurses' association within two months of the seminar on professionalism.
Psychomotor	Mrs. Thomas will draw up the correct amount of insulin in the syringe without breaking sterile technique.

occur at the time of the assessment or at a future time. The objectives dictate the content and the teaching strategies to be used. Teaching/ learning texts identify some key factors to consider when planning education for an individual or a group (Farquharson, 1995; Buchanan & Glanville, 1988; Megenity & Megenity, 1982; Rorden, 1987; Van Hoozer et al., 1987; Whitman et al., 1992). These include: creating set, reinforcement, use of examples or models, questioning, simulations, and problem-solving.

Sets, or expectations, precondition the learner to the instruction. The learner's interest is aroused and there is an expectancy for the teaching based on the objectives. A positive approach to the learning process is desired. For example, telling new nurses the reason that they need to know a unit of content on discharge planning for their job provides a positive set for learning.

Positive reinforcers strengthen learning behavior and the probability of its occurrence. Verbal praise or nonverbal communications, if linked to learning performance, can serve to motivate learning. Empirical data indicate that negative reinforcement is not effective in promoting learning.

Examples link previous knowledge to new concepts, thus encouraging understanding. Models facilitate the integration of data. Various types of models are written, verbal, or physical, for example, a model of the brain.

Questions used by the teacher focus attention on a specific concept, help to determine if more information is needed, or help to assess understanding.

A simulation is an ideal representation of a real process or occurrence. It provides the learner with the opportunity to experience an event without the threat of failure or injury to self or others. Simulations can be verbal, written, audiovisual or computer-managed. They provide excellent opportunities for learners to enhance their problem solving skills. Problem-solving as a teaching/learning strategy enables the learner to use available data to make decisions to act or obtain additional data.

TEACHING STRATEGIES/METHODOLOGIES

The actual teaching phase of the process includes many activities encompassing explaining, demonstrating, and reinforcing. If assessment and planning have been carefully done, the formal type of teaching should clearly follow. The reader is referred to teaching/learning resources referred to above for specific details of methods such as lecturing, leading group discussions, or role-playing. Implementation of the more informal teaching or coaching is less easy to specify. Much of this type of teaching follows from a sound knowledge and experience base which may almost collapse the assessment, planning, implementation, and evaluation into one function, though the elements of each are present.

Coaching a person through an illness, or taking what is foreign and fearful to the person and making it familiar and less frightening, are important responsibilities of APNs. Coaching takes great skill and understanding, not only of the condition and its trajectory, but of the person involved. In addition to information, expert nurses share ways of coping (Benner, 1984).

Competencies of the expert nurse in the teaching/coaching domain were identified by Benner (1984) and modified by Brykczynski (1989) for nurse practitioners. Competencies added to the teaching/coaching function by Brykczynski included teaching for self-care, making illness approachable and understandable, and negotiating when the client/provider priorities conflict (Fenton & Brykczynski, 1993). The educator role of the APN includes such activities as timing, assisting, eliciting, providing, negotiating, and coaching.

In timing, a patient's readiness to learn is captured. The APN creates a climate which facilitates learning. Based on an assessment of health behaviors and learning needs of the client and his/her readiness to learn, the APN provides teaching and guidance. Anticipatory guidance is provided at the appropriate level considering the age or developmental status of the client. The APN assists clients to integrate the implications of illness and recovery into their lifestyles. The APN teaches self-care, including suggesting options so clients can maximize their abilities and enjoy an optimal quality of life. Assisting clients with goal-setting for health promotion and maintenance, and establishing plans or protocols for group teaching, are APN competencies.

Eliciting an understanding of the client's interpretation of his or her illness is another skill APNs will use in teaching. People have their own understanding of wellness and what might promote or interfere with their health. Likewise, persons who become ill have their own interpretation and understanding of their condition. Nurses must incorporate this information into their teaching; sometimes myths need to be dispelled, while at other times clarification is all that is needed.

APNs provide an interpretation of the client's condition and the rationale for specific procedures. The APN provides information about the therapeutic regimes, including therapeutic actions, side effects, and instructions that will promote the optimal effects. Teaching strategies are used that are appropriate to the client's age, health problem, level of functioning, emotional needs, and other characteristics. Nurses and other health care professionals now realize that patients want to know what is being done to them and why. They need to know so they can assume some control over their lives. The expert nurse uses knowledge about the condition and the person to select the amount of information to share and the method of sharing. Choice of vocabulary is very important, so that the person understands but does not feel incompetent. Sometimes nurses must admit that they don't know the answers, and must seek other resources or share the frustration of the unknown along with the client.

In negotiating, client participation is maximized and control over his/her own care is optimized. Barriers to learning and behavior change are assessed. When the client's priorities conflict with those of the health care provider, negotiations are necessary.

Coaching is the final component of the APN's teaching/coaching role. APNs provide culturally sensitive care, making culturally avoided aspects of an illness approachable and understandable. Empirical data have shown that persons want to share their concerns about their illness, their fears about dying, and about other topics that may be socially unmentionable. The APN develops ways of determining acceptable times and places for such interactions with clients and their families. Counseling in crisis/loss/grief situations is done with referral to other health care providers as appropriate. The advanced practice nurse guides the client through emotional and developmental changes.

EVALUATION OF EFFECTIVENESS

Evaluation is inherent in nursing practice and nursing education. Assessment/evaluation is ongoing; however, documentation of the results of outcomes is necessary for the client, the APN, and the health care delivery system. To assure that such documentation is done on a regular basis, evaluation plans must be established and shared.

Evaluation plans for documenting effectiveness of nurses in advanced practice include structure, process, and outcome (Donabedian, 1980;

Hamric, 1989). Although the greatest emphasis is on evaluation of outcomes, the three elements are functionally related. Therefore, it is useful to examine all three components.

Evaluation of structure includes measures of what the APN did in relation to functions and responsibilities included in the job description. Such evaluation might include the number of classes presented to staff, students, or the public, or the teaching protocols the nurse has prepared for staff or clients. Process evaluation examines how effectively the APN is carrying out the teaching role. Self-evaluation, peer reviews, or client evaluations may be used to determine how the APN is performing the teaching function.

Within nursing, increased emphasis is being placed on outcome-based evaluation. Nurses have been very conscious of the need to have measurable objectives which focus on what the patient or learner should be able to do when they have met the objective. Based on the objectives and outcome criteria, the nurse and client determine if the teaching has been effective. Additional teaching may be done as needed. In a formal teaching situation with primarily cognitive outcomes, this evaluation can be done more explicitly than in situations where the nurse is coaching the client who is coping with a newly diagnosed chronic illness.

The focus on cost-effectiveness has moved APNs toward using outcome measures to document cost savings when clients have received education about management of their condition. Brooten et al. (1986) documented that instruction, counseling, home visits, and daily on-call availability of a hospital-based perinatal nurse specialist for a group of Low Birth Weight (LBW) infants resulted in a savings of hospital and physician charges.

As an outcome measure of the teaching of children with poorly controlled asthma by CNSs, the number of visits to the emergency room made by these children was compared to those of a control group not having such teaching by CNSs (Alexander, Younger, Cohen, & Crawford, 1988). Using Orem's Self-Care Model, the CNSs identified the self-care deficits of the children and their families and then designed teaching to help them learn self-care behaviors. The CNS group had a significant fourfold decrease from baseline in the use of the emergency room, while the changes from baseline in the control group were not statistically significant. The rate of hospitalization or length of hospitalization was not significantly changed for either group.

Outcome measures of smoking cessation and the rate and speed of return to work of adult persons who have experienced a myocardial infarction were used to determine the effectiveness of CNSs' teaching and counseling (Pozen et al., 1977). Other researchers have used compliance with therapeutic regimes and prevention of complications as outcome measures of patient education (Gurka, 1991; Linde & Janz, 1979).

CONCLUSION

Education is an important and pervasive aspect of the APN role. Assessment for learning needs is inherent in all that the nurse does, whether for an individual client, family, community, or a group of nurses or health professional colleagues. Planning and implementation of teaching/coaching are based on assessment of needs, as are other functions of the nurse. The depth of the advanced practice nurse's educational and experience knowledge base enable immediate response to identified educational needs if necessary. This expertise makes the advanced practice nurse an excellent resource for other nurses and health care providers.

REFERENCES

Alexander, J. S., Younger, R. E., Cohen, R. M., & Crawford, L. V. (1988). Effectiveness of a nurse managed program for children with chronic asthma. *Journal of Pediatric Nursing, 3,* 312–317.

Aradine, C. R., & Denyes, M. J. (1972). Activities and pressures of clinical nurse specialists. *Nursing Research, 21,* 411–418.

Benner, P. (1984). *From novice to expert.* Menlo Park, CA: Addison-Wesley.

Beyerman, K. (1988). Consultation roles of the clinical nurse specialist: A case study. *Clinical Nurse Specialist, 2,* 91–95.

Bloom, B. S. (Ed.) (1956). *Taxonomy of educational objectives.* New York: David McKay.

Brooten, D., Brown, L. P., Munro, B. H., York, R., Cohen, S., Roncoli, M., & Hollingsworth, A. (1988). Early discharge and specialist transitional care. *Image: Journal of Nursing Scholarship, 20,* 64–68.

Brooten, D., Gennaro, S., Knapp, H., Jovene, N., Brown, L., & York, R. (1991). CNS functions in early discharge of very low birthweight infants. *Clinical Nurse Specialist, 5,* 196–201.

Brooten, D., Kumar, S., Butts, P., Finkler, S., Bakewell-Sachs, S., Gibbons, A., & Delivoria-Papadopoulos, M. (1986). A randomized clinical trial of early hospital discharge and home follow-up of very low birthweight infants. *New England Journal of Medicine, 315*, 934–939.

Brykczynski, K. A. (1989). An interpretive study describing the clinical judgement of nurse practitioners. *Scholarly Inquiry for Nursing Practice: An International Journal, 3*, 75–104.

Buchanan, B. F., & Glanville, C. I. (1988). The clinical nurse specialist as educator: Process and method. *Clinical Nurse Specialist, 2*, 82–89.

Burge, S., Crigler, L., Hurth, L., Kelly, L., & Sandborn, C. (1989). Clinical nurse specialist role development: Quantifying actual practice over three years. *Clinical Nurse Specialist, 3*, 33–36.

Caffarella, R. S. (1994). *Planning programs for adult learners.* San Francisco: Jossey-Bass.

Cason, C. L., & Beck, C. M. (1982). Clinical nurse specialist role development. *Nursing and Health Care, 3*, 35–38.

Donabedian, A. (1980). *The definition of quality and approaches to its assessment: Explorations in quality assessment and monitoring.* Ann Arbor, MI: Health Administration Press.

Elder, R. G., & Bullough, B. (1990). Nurse practitioners and Clinical nurse specialists: Are the roles merging? *Clinical Nurse Specialist, 4*, 78–84.

Falvo, D. (1985). *Effective patient education: A guide to increased compliance.* Rockville, MD: Aspen.

Farquharson, A. (1995). *Teaching in practice.* San Francisco: Jossey-Bass.

Fenton, M. V. (1985). Identifying competencies of clinical nurse specialist. *Journal of Nursing Administration, 15*, 31–37.

Fenton, M. V., & Brykczynski, K. A. (1993). Qualitative distinctions and similarities in the practice of clinical nurse specialist and nurse practitioners. *Journal of Professional Nursing, 9*, 313–326.

Gift, A. D. (1992). Effectiveness of the CNS as educator and discharge planner. *Clinical Nurse Specialist, 6*, 201.

Girouard, S. A. (1996). Evaluating advanced nursing practice. In A. B. Hamric, J. A. Spross, & C. M. Hanson (Eds.), *Advanced nursing practice: An integrative approach* (pp. 569–600). Philadephia: Saunders.

Gurka, A. M. (1991). Process and outcome components of clinical nurse specialist consultation. *Dimensions of Critical Care Nursing, 10*, 169–175.

Hamric, A. B. (1989). A model for CNS evaluation. In A. B. Hamric & J. A. Spross (Eds.), *The clinical nurse specialist in theory and practice* (pp. 83–104). Philadelphia: Saunders.

Hart, C., Lekander, R., Bartels, D., & Tebbitt, B. (1987). Clinical nurse specialists: An institutional process for determining priorities. *Journal of Nursing Administration, 17*, 31–35.

Jazwiec, R. M. (1985). Learning needs assessment: A complex process. *Journal of Nursing Staff Development, 1*, 91–96.

Kelly, K. J. (Ed.) (1992). *Nursing staff development: Current competence, future focus.* Philadelphia: Lippincott.

Knowles, M., & Associates. (1984). *Andragogy in action.* San Francisco: Jossey-Bass.

Knowles, M. S. (1970). *The modern practice of adult education: Andragogy versus pedagogy.* New York: Association Press.

Linde, B., J., & Janz, N. M. (1979). Effects of a teaching program on knowledge and compliance of cardiac patients. *Nursing Research, 28,* 282–286.

Maslow, A. (1970). *Motivation and personality.* New York: Harper and Row.

Megenity, J., & Megenity, J. (1982). *Patient teaching: Theories, techniques and strategies.* Bowie, MD: Robert J. Brady.

Miller, P. J. (1992). Planning programs: Strategies for success. In K. J. Kelly (Ed.), *Nursing staff development: Current competence, future focus* (pp. 117–154). Philadelphia: Lippincott.

Narrow, B. W. (1979) *Patient teaching in nursing practice.* New York: Wiley.

Pew Health Professions Commission (1991). *Healthy America: Practitioners for 2005: An agenda for action for U. S. health professional schools.* Durham, NC: Author.

Pozen, M. N., Stechmiller, J. A. ., Harris, W. A., Smith, S., Fried, D. D., & Voight, G. C. (1977). A nurse rehabilitator's impact on patients with myocardial infarction. *Medical Care, 15,* 830–837.

Puetz, B. E. (1992). Needs assessment: The essence of staff development programs. In K. J. Kelly (Ed.), *Nursing staff development: Current competence, future focus* (pp. 97–116). Philadelphia: Lippincott.

Rankin, S. H., & Stallings, K. D. (1990). *Patient education: Issues, principles, practices.* Philadelphia: Lippincott.

Robichaud, A. M., & Hamric, A. (1986). Time documentation of clinical nurse specialist activities. *Journal of Nursing Administration, 16,* 31–36.

Rorden, J. W. (1987). *Nurses as health teachers: A practical guide.* Philadelphia: Saunders.

Simsek, H., & Heydinger, R. B. (1992, October). *A paradigm shift in the U. S. higher education system: Analysis and implications.* Paper presented at the annual meeting of the Association for the Study of Higher Education, Minneapolis, MN.

Taristano, B. J., Brophy, E. B., & Snyder, D. J. (1986). A demystification of the clinical nurse specialist role: Perceptions of clinical nurse specialists and nurse administrators. *Journal of Nursing Education, 25,* 4–9.

Van Hoozer, H. L., & Bratton, B. D. Ostmoe, P. M., Weinholtz, D., Craft, M. J., Gjerde, C., L., & Albanese, M. A. (1987). *The teaching process: Theory and practice in nursing.* Norwalk, CT: Appleton-Century-Crofts.

Whitman, N. I., Graham, B. A., Gleit, C. J., & Boyd, M. D. (1992). *Teaching in nursing practice: A professional model.* Norwalk, CT: Appleton & Lange.

Chapter 8

COMPLEMENTARY THERAPIES

Pamela J. Weiss, PhD, RN, Dipl. Ac., L.Ac

When the terms "complementary" or "alternative" therapies are used, they convey that these therapies are used in addition to the treatments of the dominant system. Increasingly, the American public is using more complementary/alternative therapies. In two recent surveys (Astin, 1998; Eisenberg et al., 1998), findings indicated that over one-third of the persons surveyed used some form of complementary/alternative therapies. Eisenberg et al. (1998) found that Americans spent over $32.7 billion on complementary therapies, with at least $12.2 billion paid for by the individual and not by third-party payers. Greater validation for these therapies was provided when the National Institutes of Health (NIH) established the Office of Alternative Medicine (OAM) in 1992. In 1998, OAM became the Center for Complementary and Alternative Medicine. Because of the increasing demand for complementary therapies, many health care plans are beginning to include some complementary therapies in the services offered. It is important that advanced practice nurses (APNs) have a general knowledge about these therapies and include some of these therapies in the care they provide. Although a number of the complementary therapies have a long tradition as part of nursing, APNs may desire to pursue additional coursework/preparation to become providers of additional therapies.

DEFINITIONS

The term "dominant health care system" is often used to distinguish care offered within the American or Western health care system from therapies associated with non-Western care systems. Western medicine or conventional medicine are terms that are commonly used to designate the dominant health system found in the United States. Other terms that are used include scientific medicine, traditional medicine, allopathic medicine, evidence-based medicine, and biomedicine. Berkenwald (1998) suggested that terms such as "scientific medicine" imply that other healing systems are not grounded in reality. The term "traditional medicine" has been used to describe many systems of medicine that have their roots in ancient cultures. Use of the term "allopathic medicine" implies that physicians are being compared to homeopathic physicians. Because of the above and other objections to numerous labels used to indicate the dominant American system of care, the term "biomedicine" will be used throughout this chapter.

Likewise, numerous terms have been used to encompass the therapies used that are not part of the biomedical system. These include unconventional medicine, unproven medicine, unorthodox medicine, nontraditional medicine, folk medicine, holistic care, alternative therapies or medicine, integrative medicine, quackery, alternative therapies/medicine, and complementary therapies/medicine. Berkenwald (1998) suggested that many of these terms mislead readers. Terms such as "unproven," "unconventional," and "unorthodox" suggest that no evidence exists supporting the efficacy of the therapies. However, a substantial historical record for the effectiveness of many therapies can be found in a multitude of cultures.

Weil and Smith (1995) coined the term "integrative medicine" to describe the combination of biomedicine and complementary therapies in the delivery of care. Integrative medicine includes the therapies of herbs, physical manipulation, and acupuncture in addition to biomedical therapies.

"Quackery" is used by some groups to designate non-biomedical therapies, as these persons believe that many therapies lack double-blind investigations to prove their efficacy. Use of the term "alternative therapies" suggests that no biomedical treatments are included in the care plan; in many instances, both biomedical and other therapies are combined to treat a health care problem.

Complementary therapies/medicine is the term frequently used throughout Europe to designate non-biomedical therapies. "Complementary therapies" is the desired term and will be used in this chapter; "therapies" and not "medicine," as many health professionals, not only physicians, administer non-biomedical therapies.

The NIH National Center for Complementary and Alternative Medicine has noted that a large number of healing resources are included under the rubric of complementary/alternative therapies. The definition for these therapies that was developed by an interdisciplinary panel is:

> Complementary medicine is a broad domain of healing resources that encompasses all health care systems, modalities, and practices and their accompanying theories and beliefs, other than those intrinsic to the politically dominant health system of a particular society or culture in a given historical period. CAM includes all such practices and ideas self-defined by their users as preventing or treating illness or promoting health and well-being. Boundaries within CAM and between the CAM domain and the domains of the dominant system are not always sharp and fixed. (Panel on Definition & Description, 1997, p. 50)

Several important elements are found in the above definition. First, what constitutes complementary therapies varies depending on the country or culture. For example, in China, Western biomedical therapies are complementary to Traditional Chinese Medicine. Secondly, as therapies gain more credence and use, they may no longer be considered complementary, but rather a part of the dominant health system. Lastly, a vast variety of therapies are encompassed under the rubric of "complementary therapies." Chez and Jonas (1998) identified more than 350 different therapies that fit within the broad domain of complementary therapies.

Complementary therapies have been classified in a variety of ways. The classification system for complementary therapies proposed by the National Center for Complementary and Alternative Medicine is found in Table 8.1. A number of these therapies, such as Therapeutic Touch and meditation, are familiar to APNs. Several texts provide detailed information about specific complementary therapies frequently used by nurses (Dossey, Keegan, Guzzetta, & Kolkmeier, 1995; Snyder & Lindquist, 1998). Fewer APNs may be familiar with other categories, particularly the systems of care. A brief overview of some of these complementary systems will be provided.

TABLE 8.1   NIH Classifications of Complementary and Alternative Medicine

Alternative Systems of Medical Practice
- Traditional Asian Medicine
- Ayurveda
- Native American Healing
- Curanderismo

Energy Medicine
- Therapeutic Touch
- Healing Touch
- Qi Gong
- Reiki

Bioelectromagnetic Systems
- Electrostimulation
- Full Spectrum Lighting
- Light Therapy

Manual Therapies
- Massage
- Acupressure
- Movement Therapies
- Reflexology
- Chiropractic
- Osteopathy
- Rolfing
- Feldenkrias

Mind-Body Therapies
- Relaxation Techniques
- Guided Imagery
- Biofeedback
- Counseling
- Prayer
- Music Therapy
- Meditation
- Humor Therapy
- Hypnosis

Diet, Nutrition, Lifestyle
- Special Diets
- Breathing Patterns
- Nutritional Supplements
- Megavitamins
- Exercise

Herbal Medicine
- Native American Herbalism
- Traditional Asian Herbalism
- European Phytochemical Herbalism

Note: Adapted from National Center for complementary and alternative medicine (1999). Available: on-line http://alt.med.od.nih.gov/nccam/what-is-cam/

COMPLEMENTARY SYSTEMS OF CARE

Advanced practice nurses provide care for persons from diverse cultures. Therefore, knowledge about some of the more common systems of care will be helpful to APNs in providing knowledgeable care. A more extensive description of systems of care can be found in a variety of texts such as *Fundamentals of Complementary and Alternative Medicine* (Micozzi, 1996). Websites are an excellent resource for the latest information about systems of care and specific therapies. A list of websites on complementary therapies is found in Table 8.2.

Complementary systems of practice range from self-care according to folk principles to care rendered in an organized health care system. The most striking factor that differentiates these systems of care/therapies from biomedicine is that persons are viewed from a holistic perspective. These systems contain specialized diagnostic methods and treatments that are individualized to each patient based not only on the symptoms assessed, but also on the underlying strengths and weaknesses of the patient. Basic elements of some of these systems will be described.

Advanced practice nurses who learn other therapies, and particularly other systems of care, will most often use these therapies within the existing biomedical system of care. It is interesting to speculate about

TABLE 8.2   Websites for content related to complementary therapies

Acupuncture	http://www.acupuncture.com
Holistic Nursing	http://www.ahna.org
National Center for Complementary & Alternative medicine (NCCAM)	http://altmed.od.nih.gov/oam
MedWeb: Alternative Medicine	http:\\www.gen.emory.edu/medweb/medweb.altmed.html
Andrew Weil	http://www.weil.com
International Society for the Study of Subtle Energies	http://vitalenergy.com/issseem/index.html
American Herbalists Guild	http:\\www.health.net/pan/pa/herbalmedicine/ahg/index.html
Rosenthal Center for Legal and Regulatory Information	http:\\cpmcnet.columbia.edu/dept/rosenthal/AM_legal.html
Complementary Traditional Medicine	http://utmednet.org/im/gen/wellness/.html

how APNs would function within other systems of care, such as Traditional Chinese Medicine or Native American care.

Traditional Oriental Medicine/Traditional Chinese Medicine

Traditional Chinese Medicine (TCM) is a sophisticated set of many systematic techniques and methods, including acupuncture, herbal medicine, acupressure, qigong, and oriental massage. TCM has an extensive history and was widely practiced centuries before many of the biomedical therapies were evaluated. The philosophical basis for TCM is yin and yang. According to Ergil (1996), these two concepts express the idea of opposing, but complementary phenomena that exist in a state of dynamic equilibrium. Both are always present.

Traditional Chinese physicians often use the elements of yin and yang to organize information gained during an examination. The most striking characteristic of TCM is the emphasis on diagnosing disturbances of qi, or vital energy, in health and disease. Diagnosis in TCM involves the classical procedures of observation, listening, questioning, and palpation, including feeling pulse quality and sensitivity of body parts.

Acupuncture, the most well known TCM therapy, involves stimulating specific anatomic points in the body for therapeutic purposes. Puncturing the skin with a needle is the usual method, but practitioners also use heat, pressure, friction, suction, or impulses of electromagnetic energy to stimulate points. In 1997, the NIH held a consensus conference on acupuncture (NIH, 1997). Participants concluded that acupuncture is a proven effective treatment for adult postoperative nausea and the nausea and vomiting associated with chemotherapy. Use of acupuncture has a high probability of being effective in reducing perioperative dental pain, reducing the nausea associated with pregnancy, and reducing the discomfort associated with menstrual cramps.

Herbal preparations are another key component of TCM. Over 5,767 herbs, minerals, and animal parts that are used in treating persons are contained in the *Encyclopedia of Traditional Chinese Medicinal Substances* that was published in 1977 by the Jiangsu College of New Medicine.

Learning TCM requires a significant commitment of time. The formalized training program consists of 2250 hours of study. Certification is granted by the National Commission of Acupuncture and Oriental Medicine. Specific licensure to practice TCM or acupuncture is required in 38 states.

Ayurvedic Medicine

Ayurveda is the world's oldest system of natural medicine. It had its origins over 5000 years ago in India. This system provides an integrated approach for preventing and treating illness through lifestyle interventions and natural therapies. Ayurvedic medicine is based on the belief that all disease begins with an imbalance or stress in an individual's consciousness. *Vyaadhi* (disease) is due to an imbalance of the three fundamental elements of the body: *vata, pitta,* and *kapha.* These three elements are combinations of space, air, light, water, and earth. Ayurvedic medicine has been divided into eight branches: internal medicine; pediatrics; diseases related to pathogens, evil spirits, etc.; problems related to eyes, ears, nose, throat, and dentistry; surgery; insect bites and poisons; diseases of advancing age; and, gynecology and obstetrics. Drugs specific to Ayurvedic medicine are used; these drugs are made from vegetable and mineral raw materials.

The research base for use of Ayurvedic medicine is increasing. Positive outcomes for meditative and yoga postures have been documented in Indian and Western literature. Published studies have documented reduction in cardiovascular disease risk factors such as blood pressure, cholesterol, and reaction to stress in persons who practice Ayurvedic methods (Dogra, Grover, Kumar, & Aneja, 1994). Laboratory and clinical evidence on Ayurvedic herbal preparations have shown them to be potentially beneficial in preventing and treating certain cancers and infectious diseases and in promoting health and treating aging (Prasad, Perry, & Chan, 1993).

Preparation in Ayurvedic medicine can be obtained in the United States. Westbrook University in Portland, Maine, provides opportunities for pursuing of master's and doctoral degrees in Ayurveda medicine. Also available is a 600-hour diploma course.

Native American Indian Community-Based Care

Healing practices vary across Native American communities. However, a number of rituals and practices are practiced in many communities: sweating and purging, which are usually done in a sweat lodge; use of herbal remedies gathered from the surrounding environment; and, shamanic healing, involving naturalistic and personalistic healing practices. Tribes such as the Lakota and Dineh (Navajo) also use practices such as the medicine wheel, sacred hoop, and the sing. The latter is a healing ceremony that lasts 2 to 9 days and is guided by a highly skilled specialist called a singer.

Formal research about the healing ceremonies and herbal medicines used by Native American healers and holy people is almost nonexistent. However, Native Americans have a strong faith in the efficacy of these therapies. Sanchez, Plawecki and Plawecki (1996) provide information about plants and herbs commonly used by many tribes in the United States. Native American doctors who are knowledgeable about these complex ceremonies have reported cures of heart disease, diabetes, thyroid conditions, cancer, skin rashes, and asthma.

Curanderismo

Curanderismo is one of the folk systems of care used in a number of Latin American cultures. This folk system of medicine includes two distinct components: a humoral model for classifying activity, food, drugs, and illness, and a classification of illnesses and remedies. In the humoral component of Curanderismo, objects can be classified as having qualitative (not literal) characteristics of hot or cold and dry or moist. According to this theory, keeping a balance of hot and cold is essential to maintaining good health. Thus, a good meal will contain both hot and cold foods. A person with a hot disease will be given cold remedies, and vice versa. A person who is exposed to cold when excessively hot may take cold and become ill.

The second component, classification of folk illnesses, is used throughout Mexico and by many persons of Hispanic descent who live in the United States. Studies have shown that as many as 32% to 96% of Mexican-American households (more frequent in the less Americanized communities) recognize folk illnesses and receive treatment for these illnesses (Trotter, 1985). Although no formal effectiveness studies have been done to determine the efficacy of these practices, the wide use of these practices necessitates that research be conducted.

Other Systems

Two other systems of care which are gaining popularity in the United States are homeopathy and naturopathy. Homeopathy and naturopathy have a long history of use both in the United States and in other countries.

*Homeopathy**

This system of care is primarily used by lay practitioners in the United States. According to the Institute of Alternative Futures, "homeopathy combines a set of standardized medicinal remedies with sophisticated analysis of the patients' `constitutional factors,' which is used to personalize the selection and dosing of a remedy to each individual." (p. 6-1). Homeopathic remedies, which are made from naturally occurring plant, animal, and mineral substances, are recognized and regulated by the Food and Drug Administration (FDA) but in a different manner than other medications. These substances are manufactured by established pharmaceutical companies. Homeopathy is used to treat acute and chronic health problems as well as to prevent disease and promote health.

Naturopathy

According to Pizzorno (1996), naturopathic medicine is a way of life. It is not associated with any one therapy, but rather with a philosophy of life which supports the body healing itself when it is given the opportunity and the person lives within the laws of nature. Great diversity exists in naturopathy, with some practitioners adhering to the use of natural cures such as diet and lifestyle modification, while other practitioners incorporate many therapies from conventional medicine. Thus, the therapies used are diverse and can include natural therapies including botanical medicine, clinical nutrition, homeopathy, acupuncture, TCM, hydrotherapy, and naturopathic manipulative therapies with modern medical diagnostic science and standards of care. Research at naturopathic institutes is of recent origin, but a substantial body of published findings on naturopathic therapies has been published.

PREPARATION FOR USING COMPLEMENTARY THERAPIES

Changes in the health care system are affecting practitioners providing complementary therapies. Health provider organizations are seeking ways

---

*Although research on homeopathy is increasing, results are inconclusive at this time.

to verify training and expertise of practitioners so as to provide safe and effective care. Since the majority of APN educational programs do not include extensive content on complementary therapies, APNs desiring to become proficient in the administration of specific complementary therapies will need to seek continuing education and certification programs. The length of the program will vary depending on the nature of the therapy. For example, to become a certified massage therapist requires 500 hours of training. Certification for healing touch, which includes Therapeutic Touch, is a multi-level program. Levels I and II each consists of 15 hours of instruction whereas Level III is approximately 6 to 12 months in length and consists of two, 30-hour sections.

Accrediting agencies and associations exist for a number of the complementary therapies. The accrediting agencies specify the content of educational programs. Other organizations offer certification examinations. As the popularity of complementary therapies increases, more states are increasing their regulation of these therapies so as to protect the public from fraud. State regulations may require certification or licensure for persons to administer certain therapies (Beck, 1996). It is important for APNs to become familiar with the educational preparation/licensure requirements in specific states.

There are many complementary therapies that are within the domain of nursing. Some of these therapies are relaxation techniques, exercise, massage, biofeedback, imagery, presence, Therapeutic Touch, humor, assisting with lifestyle changes, and helping sustain family and significant other relationships (Dossey et al., 1995; Snyder & Lindquist, 1998). Advanced practice nurses can incorporate these into their practice without additional certification.

INCLUSION OF COMPLEMENTARY THERAPIES IN PRACTICE

A number of surveys (Arcury, Bernard, Jordan, & Cook, 1996; Astin, 1998; Eisenberg et al., 1998; Harris, 1996; Kristoffersen, Atkin, & Shenfield, 1996; Risberg, Lund, Weist, Kaasa, & Wilsgaard, 1998) have explored the extent to which persons are using complementary therapies. The smallest percentage of use was by cancer patients; only 17.4%–27.3% reported use of these therapies (Risberg et al., 1998). This is in contrast to persons with arthritis; 92% reported use of complementary therapies (Arcury et al., 1996). In the national surveys conducted by Eisenberg et al. (1998) and Astin (1998), the reported rates of use of complementary therapies were 46.3% and 40%, respectively. These statistics may be a conservative estimate about the use of complementary therapies, as persons may be reluctant to indicate that they use non-biomedical therapies. The rapid growth of nutrition centers that sell herbs and nutraceuticals is indicative of the wide use of complementary therapies. The most common therapies used by persons surveyed were massage, herbs, relaxation techniques, spiritual and meditation practices, megavitamins, and chiropractic care.

Eisenberg and colleagues (1998) reported that 96% of the persons using complementary therapies consulted their medical doctor for the same condition. What is startling is that only 38.5% disclosed to their physician that they were using other therapies. Because complementary therapies can enhance or interfere with the effects of biomedical treatments, it is important for the APN to obtain information about a patient's use of these therapies. Merely asking a patient if he/she is using complementary therapies may not elicit this information, as the term itself may be unfamiliar to the person. The APN must ask the patient about use of specific therapies such as massage, meditation, herbs, neutraceuticals, or homeopathic preparations.

When the APN identifies that a patient is using a specific complementary therapy, this information needs to be considered when prescribing conventional therapies/medications. If the APN is not familiar with the therapy, information will need to be obtained. Websites noted in Table 8.2 are a readily available resource. A reference describing common herbal preparations is also beneficial. Developing a network of colleagues who are knowledgeable about specific therapies is also valuable. Also, knowing persons who are able providers of therapies will allow the APN to make referrals. When acting as a resource for patients as they make decisions about use of complementary therapies, Eisenberg (1997) recommended discussing the patient's preferences and expectations, reviewing safety issues, helping the patient find a qualified provider, and suggesting that the patient keep a journal about the efficacy of the therapy.

Nurses' knowledge about complementary therapies varies. In a survey of APNs in the New England area, Bacon (1998) found that nurses had the most knowledge about therapeutic touch and the least knowledge about Reiki. Respondents perceived acupuncture to be the most helpful modality and Reiki to be the least helpful. Nurses surveyed had little knowledge about herbal products. These findings support the need for APN educational programs to include more information about complementary therapies. This content needs to include the most recent research findings on specific complementary therapies. Research on complementary therapies is growing; providing patients and professional colleagues with information about the scientific basis for therapies will help to gain acceptance for these therapies.

Nurses have a tradition of approaching patients from a holistic perspective, with healing and health promotion being primary care outcomes. Thus, an APN's practice would be incomplete if administration of complementary therapies were not included in the armamentarium of therapies offered to patients. These therapies can range from those as simple as hand massage to more complex ones such as biofeedback, acupuncture, or aromatherapy. Often additional preparation may be needed before an APN can safely administer these therapies.

CURRICULAR IMPLICATIONS

Currently, many curricula for advanced practice nurses do not include content on complementary and alternative therapies. In a survey of APN programs, Rauckhorst (1997) found that the majority (63%) of the 118 programs responding did not include content on complementary therapies in their curricula. Forty-two programs noted that they did include this content. Obstacles noted for not including content on complementary therapies were objections from the medical community, limited opportunities to practice the therapies, lack of time in the curricula, and lack of faculty expertise. Providing APN students with content about complementary therapies promotes culturally sensitive and holistic care and increases the self-care options for patients. It is also important that APNs have knowledge about the research that supports the use of specific therapies.

Including content on complementary therapies does present challenges to faculty. It may be difficult to obtain faculty who have expertise in therapies such as homeopathy, TCM, Ayurvedic medicine, and herbs. Finding time within an already full curriculum is another challenge. However, the increasing diversity of patients served, the increasing number of Americans using and requesting complementary therapies, and the publics desire for holistic care mandates that APN curricula include sufficient content on complementary therapies.

REFERENCES

Arcury, T. A., Bernard, S. L., Jordan, J. M., & Cook, H. L. (1996). Gender and ethnic differences in alternative and conventional arthritis remedy use among community-dwelling rural adults with arthritis. *Arthritis Care & Research, 9,* 384–90.

Astin, J. A. (1998). Why patients use alternative medicine. *Journal of the American Medical Association, 279,* 1548–1553.

Bacon, M. M. (1997). Nurse practitioner's views and knowledge of herbal medicine and alternative healing methods. *University of Lowell MA,* Vol. 35-04, Page 0996. 0044 Pages. Dissertation Abstracts MAI 35/04, p. 96.

Beck, R. L. (1996). An overview of state alternative healing practices law. *Alternative Therapies, 2,* 31–33.

Berkenwald, A. D. (1998). In the name of medicine. *Annals of Internal Medicine, 128,* 246–250.

Chez, R. Z., & Jonas, W. (1998). One kind of medicine or many? The view from NIH. *Contemporary Ob/Gyn, 43* (2), 123–124, 129–130, 133–134.

Dacher, E. S. (1996). Post modern medicine. *Journal of Alternative and Complementary Medicine, 2,* 531–537.

Dogra, J., Grover, N., Kumar, P., & Aneja, N. (1994). Indigenous free radical scavenger MAK 4 and 5 in angina pectoris. Is it only a placebo? *Journal of Associated Physicians of India, 42,* 466–467.

Dossey, B. M., Keegan, L., Guzzetta, C. E., & Kolkmeir, L. G. (1995). *Holistic nursing: A handbook for practice.* Gaithersburg, MD: Aspen.

Eisenberg, D. M. (1997). Advising patients who seek alternative therapies. *Annals of Internal Medicine, 127,* 61–69.

Eisenberg, D. M., Davis, R. B., Ettner, S. L., Appel, S., Wilkey, S., Van Rompay, M., & Kessler, R. C. (1998). Trends in alternative medicine use in the United States, 1990–1997. *JAMA, 280,* 1569–1575.

Ergil, K. V. (1996). Chinas traditional medicine. In S. Micozzi (Ed.), *Fundamentals of complementary and alternative medicine* (pp. 185–223). New York: Churchill Livingstone.

Harris, B. S. (1996). *Use of alternative treatments of active duty Air Force personnel.* Unpublished master's thesis. Uniformed Services University of Health Sciences (USUHS). Naval Medicinal Comman, National Capital; Region, Bethesda, MD.

Institute for Alternative Futures. (1998). *The future of complementary and alternative approaches (CCAs) in U.S. health care.* Alexandria, VA: NCMIC Insurance Company.

Kristoffersen, S. S., Atkin, P. A., & Shenfield, G. M. (1996). Uptake of alternative medicine. *The Lancet, 347,* 9006.

NIH Consensus Statement. (1997). Acupuncture. November 3–5, 1998.

Panel on definition and description, CAM research methodology. (1997). Defining and describing complementary and alternative medicine. *Alternative Therapies, 2*(2), 49–57.

Pizzorno, J. E. (1996). Naturopathic medicine. In S. Micozzi (Ed.), *Fundamentals of complementary and alternative medicine* (pp. 163–181). New York: Churchill Livingstone.

Prasad, M. L., Parry, P., & Chan, C. (1993). Ayurvedic agents produce differential effects on murine and human melanoma cells in vitro. *Nutrition and Cancer, 20,* 79–86.

Rauckhorst, L. (1997). Integration of complementary therapies in the nurse practiioner curriculum. *Clinical Excellence for Nurse Practitioners, 1,* 257–265.

Risberg, T., Lund, E., Wist, E., Kaasa, S., & Wilsgaard, T. (1998). Cancer patients' use of non-proven therapy: A 5-year follow up study. *Journal of Clinical Oncology, 16,* 6–12.

Sanchez, T. R., Plawecki, J. A., & Plawecki, H. M. (1996). The delivering of culturally sensitive health care to Native Americans. *Holistic Nursing, 14,* 295–307.

Snyder, M. & Lindquist, R. (Eds.) (1998). *Complementary and alternative therapies in nursing.* New York: Springer Publishing Company.

Trotter, R. T. (1985). Folk medicine in the Southwest: myths and medical facts. *Postgraduate Medicine, 78,* 167–179.

Weil, A., & Smith, H. (1995). Roots of healing: the new medicine. *Alternative Therapies in Health & Medicine, 1* (2), 46–52.

Chapter **9**

CONSULTATION IN ADVANCED PRACTICE NURSING

Deborah R. Monicken, RN, MS, CRRN, CS

Consultation is an important area of practice for any Advanced Practice Nurse (APN) whether functioning primarily as a Clinical Nurse Specialist (CNS), Nurse Practitioner (NP), Certified Nurse-Midwife (CNM), or Certified Registered Nurse Anesthetist (CRNA). The utilization of consultation can help the APN's growth and value. In order to better understand the utility of this function of the APN, this chapter will explore the parameters of consultation, discuss the preparation for and development of the consultant's abilities, and review the consultant's function in multiple consultation nursing settings and in the context of a practice model. In addition, issues surrounding the ethics, power, and utility of consultation will be addressed.

PARAMETERS OF CONSULTATION

The activities of the APN in the area of consultation are well documented in the literature (Badger, 1988; Barron, 1989; Noll, 1987). Noll notes

149

that the primary practice role of the CNS should be that of an internal consultant. Certainly, consultation could be considered a primary vehicle for the dissemination of an APN's expertise. However, internal consultation is no longer the primary avenue of consultation for the APN. In the current economies of health care, external consultation is not only an economic necessity, but also is an opportunity for the evolution of the APN role. In the recent austerity of this economy, for the business that has supported the APN role, diversity of the APN's activities in conjunction with consultation can be as much of an economic imperative as a lucrative venture.

Caplan (1970) defines consultation as "a process of interaction between two professional persons—the consultant, who is a specialist, and the consultee, who invokes the consultant's help" (p.19). Consultation can be described by the type of client served, the type of activities requested in the consultation, the method of consultation (formal or informal) provided, and the relationship of the consultant to the organization (internal vs. external). Consultation is categorized in four ways: 1) client-centered case consultation; 2) consultee-centered case consultation; 3) program-centered administrative consultation; and 4) consultee-centered administrative consultation (Caplan).

Consultation requires much planning prior to the actual consultation meeting. Lippitt and Lippitt (1978) provide a six-phase guide to consultation which has been utilized in a variety of consultation situations (See Table 9.1). In practice, Caplan's client-centered consultation is often accomplished using an informal approach in phases I and II of this process. This commonly occurs because of the casual nature and frequency of this type of consult in a nurse to APN interaction. Though this informal approach can have the advantages of being time-saving and educational, Manian and Janssen (1996) warn that the consultant (and client's care) can be vulnerable to incomplete information/examination, especially if the consult is of a complex nature. The informal approach can lead to the provision of erroneous recommendations, and these recommendations may be documented in the health record, which could create future legal complications. Likewise, there is also the concern of lost fee-for-service income/documentation of workload.

According to Edlund, Hodges, and Poteet (1987), a consultation can be requested by informal (verbal contact) or formal (written contract) technique. Though both approaches are acceptable, this author finds that the consultee, particularly in client-centered issues, is better able to organize concerns when a formal approach is used. In Caplan's three other types of consultation, while informal discussions are initially essential

TABLE 9.1   Phases of Consultation

Phase	Description of Activity
I. Contact and entry change,	Make contact, identify needs and readiness to and discuss possibility of working together.
II. Formulating a contract and establishing a helping relationship	Outline desired outcomes, assign jobs/responsibilities, and formulate time framework and accountability
III. Problem identification and diagnostic analysis	Problem analysis, data collection, evaluation of forces working for or against any movement, and considerations of the readiness to change
IV. Goal-setting and planning	Project goals and plan action/involvement
V. Taking action and cycling feedback	Successful action taken based on expertise, evaluation, and feedback for necessary person, revision of actions, and acquisition of additional resources
VI. Contract completion, continuity, support, and termination	Designing continued support systems to assure continued success and planning termination time frame and resident expertise

Note: Adapted from *The Consulting Process in Action* (pp. 9–26) by G. Lippitt and R. Lippitt, 1978, La Jolla, CA: University Associates, Inc.

to understanding issues, ultimately, a formal contract should be written informally.

Actually, these first two phases of consultation are the ones that should be most emphasized if there is to be consultee collaboration and accountability. In some consulting situations, with breakdown in this process, the consultee (i.e., other nurse) abdicates involvement, giving the APN full responsibility for problem identification and resolution. When this happens, the consultee relinquishes any accountability, and the consultant becomes a direct caregiver. This type of situation is a problem for two reasons: 1) the consultant can not assume 24-hour accountability/availability, and 2) the consultee does not expand his/her knowledge and expertise for the future management of the problem.

In most other types of consultation, the phases in consultation will have more formality. As demonstrated in Figure 9.1, an organization may realize greater impact by having the APN act through a consultee-centered consultation (training of staff to do the work) than in a client-centered consultation (direct care).

In a true consultation relationship, Caplan (1970) notes that the consultant bears no direct responsibility for assuring that a recommended action is taken with a client. Instead, the action taken is the responsibility of the consultee. The consultee has the option of accepting or reject-

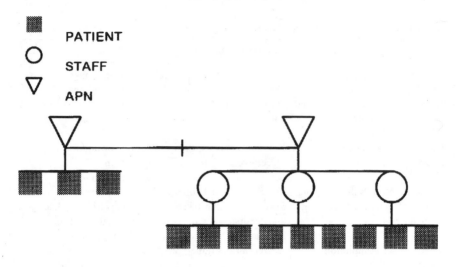

■ PATIENT

○ STAFF

▽ APN

Direct Care Model   **Consultative Care Model**

FIGURE 9.1   Comparison of the amount of expert patient care delivered by an
APN using a direct are model versus a consultative care model.

ing the advice given by the consultant. This definition leaves the accountability for the implementation of the recommendations with the
consultee.

The APN who elects to function as a consultant in this fashion must
respect the confines of a consultant's practice and the authority it assigns to others. It must be understood that though the consultant's approach provides for potential change in a client or consultee, change is
not a certainty unless it is embraced by the consultee. Some nursing
administrators may want to hold the consultant, not consultee, accountable for implementing recommendations. Expectations for the implementation of a consultant's recommendations must be clearly defined by
administration, and the activities must be understood by both the consultant and the consultee. In some institutions, APNs take a more accountable role in internal consultation. This economically has definite
advantages, and may be accomplished through measures such as continuous improvement, competency-based education, and/or standards of
care. While this approach can assure an early implementation of a consultant's efforts, it may be a short-lived change once the APN leaves if
the consultee does not embrace the change. If the APN is to be held

accountable, the APN should assure some administrative authority, either personally or in collaboration with a designated administrator. All consults, whether formal or informal, should contractually address the elements of expectations, purpose, time frame, remuneration, and need for final reports (Edlund et al., 1987). These elements need to be agreed upon by the consultant and consultee, and should be precisely stated in a document.

In recent health care trends, clients are more involved in their own care, and Alvarez (1992) points out that increasingly the client and/or family are the direct recipients of the consultant's input. This implies a greater client-controlled practice and an elimination of the "middleman" (consultee). If a consultant accepts this type of practice, expectations should be clearly outlined. For a client considering "care options" (i.e. second opinions), the APN consultant should render only recommendations. Services are provided only if the individual seeks the consultant's care.

APN PREPARATION FOR CONSULTATION

Consultation is a function into which the individual APN must evolve. It is based on the APN's knowledge, experience, and confidence. The beginning APN will generally first serve in the area of direct practice and client-centered consultations. Holt (1984) describes an evolution of development, with many of the areas of consultation occurring much later in the professional development of the APN. Certainly, the beginning APN will need time in the application of newly acquired skills to be recognized as competent by others and, personally, will need to have the confidence to provide expert consultation.

To prepare to function as a consultant, the APN must have knowledge in the areas of consultation and nursing process; a theoretical knowledge about systems, change, and adult learning; and a background in problem solving, conflict resolution, communication, and group process (Barron, 1989). Also, the consultant will need to develop abilities in self-awareness, interpersonal skills, time management, priority setting, and an ability to listen and identify areas of influence (Barron, 1989; Ulschak & Snow-Antle, 1990). A background in administration, leadership, and organizational structures, along with transcultural concepts (Leininger,

1988) is also essential. People and society are no longer homogeneous. Rather, people are as diverse as their knowledge, travels, and experiences. Culturally sensitive recommendations for each situation may be the measure of a consultant's success. Many of the aforementioned areas can not be provided solely through academic preparation or practice. There is a maturation that occurs with time, experiential opportunities, research and clinical trials.

How the APN consultant evolves is dependent on the definition and parameters of the client group, the framework of the consultant's practice, and the inherent rewards for maintaining consultation as a function of the APN practice. Over time, consultation should demonstrate growth, diversity, and mentorship as the practice is refined.

In early years of practice, the APN may remain in a consultation area where the parameters are ones of a defined client group with specific, known problems. The APN should always retain this client-oriented consultation in that it serves as a laboratory for the development of new knowledge. However, as the consultant's practice evolves, the definition of "client" should change to represent groups of patients, staff, or organizations. This is both economical and growth-producing.

The use of the Intervention Model developed by McEvoy and Egan (1979) is a very effective framework for developing the consultant's practice. This model helps the consultant identify commonalties of a population and test interventions to promote reliable outcomes. In doing this, a consultant can move from a client/consultee-specific practice to a more group-related model of practice as seen in program development and administration-centered consultation. The intervention model provides a systematic way for the consultant to collect and analyze information while looking for characteristics and trends about that population. This author has utilized this model in external consultation to help the consultee better delineate the real issues instead of describing a case-by-case scenario.

ANP CONSULTATION IN PRACTICE

In practice, the difficulties of consultation stem from the restrictions in time, parameters of focus, and limited control. The consultant needs to assure a careful preconsult preparation and ask these questions:

1) What is needed?
2) Why is it needed? (What has happened or changed that created the need?)
3) What has been tried?
4) What outcome is desired?
5) What outcome is reasonable?
6) What is the time frame?
7) What are the obstacles/resources to achieving the outcome?
8) What areas/options of change are comfortable/uncomfortable?
9) Who is important to the process?
10) What are the limits/boundaries of the consultation?

Also, in this preparation, the APN should do the following:

1) *Become familiar with the client, organization and environment.* This can be accomplished by reading the philosophy statements, procedures, and models of care of the organization, and by getting descriptions of the locale and other demographics. In client care, one might explore a client's finances, environment, etc. to assure a realistic plan of care that the client is likely to accomplish (Larsen, Risor, & Putnam, 1997).

2) *Identify a primary contact in the organization* and ensure that the individual has the ability to access needed information and has the authority to carry out the recommendations. If there are other parties involved, these should be identified. There are no greater obstacles to a plan than those that have been left out of the process.

3) *Be honest about the consultant role and the expectations about what is to be accomplished.* Know whether recommendations are to be treated as suggestions or mandates. State your limitations as a consultant whether these be due to expertise, conflict of interest or administrative restrictions. Stay within the confines of what has been requested. If other issues are identified, these can be noted if they impact the area of the consult, but they should not be acted on unless acceptable to the consultee.

4) *Allow adequate time to accomplish the work* required for the consultation. In client-based consultation, allow at least 1–2 hours for the initial visit. Subsequent follow-up can be shortened to 5–15 minutes. Consultation to an organization will vary in time depending on the size and complexity of the organization and its issues. Time should be allotted for the preparation and the evaluation components as well as the actual visit.

5) *Know why the consult was requested* and whether it is related to a

need for change. Continue to keep the client focused on a defined area.

6) *Respect the client and consultee:* Their knowledge of the problem and their ideas for the practical solutions are essential for the accomplishment of the recommendations.

7) *Know when to leave.* There are two reasons for leaving: completion of the consult, and disregard for the recommendations. If recommendations are not followed and if a comfortable compromise is not reached, the consultant can be of no value, and the consultant should terminate the contract. On the other hand, in many cases, the clients have embraced the recommendations and are functioning well with them. The best consultation outcomes occur when consultants hears their own recommendations being verbalized by the client who expresses a sense of ownership. This is the best of all changes that can be made by a consultant and is evidence of completion.

Depending on the type of consultation, the consultant can assume a variety of behaviors. Lippitt and Lippitt (1978) describe a continuum of consultant behaviors which require the consultant to be either more directive or more nondirective. The consultant assumes a greater leadership role where a more directive behavior is needed. Lippitt and Lippitt's eight consultant behaviors are: 1) Objective observer/reflector, 2) Process counselor, 3) Fact finder, 4) Alternative identifier, 5) Linker, Joint problem solver, 6) Trainer education, 7) Information expert, and 8) Advocate.

The amount of the consultant's directive behavior increases as one moves toward the latter behaviors. By correlating the APN activities with the Lippitt and Lippitt (1978) model, Beyerman (1988) found that the consulting nurse most often used the behaviors of process counselor, fact finder, informational expert, and advocate. Byerman did not contrast these behaviors with the consultant's years of experience or level of expertise (Benner, 1984). It would be interesting to consider if these behaviors varied with the consultant's level of expertise, the critical nature or priority of the problem, and/or the professional characteristics of the consultant and consultee.

Whether involved in a client or consultee consultation, an important element to the consultation process is understanding the organization. Ulshak and Snow-Antle (1990) describe a "CPR+F Model" representing the organization's purpose, roles, and feedback in communication and commitment with the organization's environment (trends, regulatory bodies, licensing groups, vendors, and professional groups) encompassing the entire model. Using the "CPR+F Model," the consultant can look at what Ulshak and Snow-Antle call the "culture" of the organization.

The consultant must understand these elements of the organization in order to know its real working layers. For example, though a similar problem might exist at two hospitals, the solutions may be different because one is a rural hospital and the other is urban. Likewise, there may be different regulations from state to state, thereby dictating a different recommendation. This information is critical to the types of recommendations made and their success. What might be essential elements to one organization may be impractical novelties in another. This knowledge is essential whether one is working within or outside of the organization.

An APN may be an internal (person inside the organization) or external (person outside the organization) consultant. Generally an internal consultant has been hired to manage ongoing issues (i.e. specific client population) that have a high prevalence and/or require long-term management. Norwood (1998a) notes that an external consultant is considered "for one of four reasons: 1) to acquire human resources, 2) to secure cost savings, 3) to ensure objectivity, or 4) to address political considerations in a problem situation" (pg. 44).

Edlund et al. (1987) describe several advantages/disadvantages to each type of consultant. Advantages of the internal consultant include: 1) being less likely to be viewed by staff as an agent of administration, 2) knowing the system's issues better, and 3) functioning better in a client or consultee consultation because of availability and follow-up. In contrast to this position, however, Lippitt and Lippitt (1978) believe that an internal consultant is viewed as being on a more subordinate level to administration, is therefore viewed by staff as an agent of administration. Edlund et al. (1987) do note that the internal consultant is more likely to be perceived as having less ability, credibility, and power. In practice, this author has found that the day-to-day presence of an internal consultant can reinforce certain practices, ensure the consultant's availability to manage changes, and provide immediate alternatives. In terms of the perceived limitations in authority or ability of the internal consultant, these issues may be based more in the person than the position.

An external consultant is often perceived as having greater administrative sanction, more knowledge, easier access to information sources, and fewer preconceived ideas about a situation. The external consultant can often be an impetus for change and, having no long-term investment, can be the "scape goat" of staff anxieties about the change, which relieves the permanent administration of the rancor (Harris, 1995). However, that same consultant has to gain the trust of staff, spend more time gaining knowledge about the system, and may still have diminished long-term effects, especially in a client or consultee consultation (Edlund et al., 1987).

It is difficult involving an external consultant in direct client care in that there is not the staff interface or day-to-day follow-up. If an APN provides external consultation on client care, such as in a workshop, it may be practical to contract for an assessment opportunity to review the clinical setting and a post-education practicum with staff to model care expectations.

As possibly the best of all alternatives, Ulshak and Snow-Antle (1990) suggest that the internal and external consultants work together. To utilize this approach, the external consultant should provide the internal consultant with increased opportunities to participate in the planning, implementation, and educational process. The external consultant should work to enhance the organization's perception of the internal consultant's expertise and authority. This approach certainly enhances the probability of long-term impact. The external consultant should contract for the time that will be required for additional meetings, coordination, and correspondence if this type of consultation is considered.

The APN may become involved in any of these consultant activities. Not knowing what elements to consider about a prospective consultation can result in unanticipated consequences. For instance, a problem area may be short-lived, and the internal consultant loses a position. There may be a history of personal agendas or insufficient support for past efforts on a problem, and the consultant will be unable to change this trend. Norwood (1998b) suggests caution when an organization seems inflexible, lacks openness, and/or lacks a commitment to the issue.

The organization, being a part of that culture, may not be mindful of the parameters of its issues. The APN must often guide the discussion and even prepare the organization for further inquiry in order to assure a consultation effort that is effective for all. Shelley (1994) suggests the "why, what, and how of working with a consultant" (p. 272) when an organization is considering a consultant. The following elements can help the APN clarify which type of consultation will be most beneficial when working with an organization on a given situation:

1) Clarity of the issue;
2) Confusion, politics, and contradictions surrounding the issue;
3) Prevalence of the issue;
4) Needs of the issue for ongoing management;
5) Existence/availability/preparation/necessity of resources over time;
6) Perceptions of indigenous expertise;

7) Immediacy of the situation; and
8) Cost.

Often, the APN is best able to screen these elements, because these exist within his/her area of expertise and the APN will have a history of past management approaches with these very issues.

MARKETING THE APN FOR CONSULTATION

On a direct care client consultation, with the health market increasingly conscious about the use of money in referrals outside of primary care, the industry has developed specific guidelines for client management. This not only helps to standardize care, but also acts as a screen for when to refer a client (Jacobs, 1997). The APN needs to become a participant in the development of these guidelines, whether on an organizational or national level, to assure that the utility of the APN consultant is incorporated into the plan.

Further, the APN needs to rethink the consumer market, as many health care corporations consolidate, thus having a large number and variety of health care services within one organization. The APN who is an internal consultant in these organizations should look at ways to expand services by promoting his/her expertise to such areas as continuity of care, standardization of care, and standardization of staff/client education throughout all these multiple services. Also, as noted earlier, there is also the opportunity for the APN to make the APN services available by marketing through the organization as an external consultant. This can help to promote the organization as a leader in health care as well as recoup the cost of retaining the internal APN consultant (Anderson, 1985; Malone, 1989).

The opportunities are growing for the APN in external consultation, from areas such as providing specialty education, program development and client care to offering expert witness/legal consultant services (McElhaney & Beare, 1998). It is important that the APN be prepared to promote his/herself to this market. Norwood (1998b) states that the APN consultant needs a stated area of expertise, recent history of consultation and clinical practice in that area of expertise, and a compatibility with the organization. Other issues that will be sought will be qualifications, references, and cost of services (Furlow & Higman, 1995). One may even be asked for a pre-interview and a proposal for the project.

If hiring is probable, it is incumbent on the APN and organization to establish certain expectations about the project. This should include role expectations, time management plan, cost/remuneration (be sure to discuss things like support staff, travel, supplies, accommodations), contact/administrative support, informational access, outcome expectations, and finally, interim and final report/interview plans (Furlow & Higman, 1995) . Norwood (1998b) encourages the creation of a partnership with someone in the organization, a preparation of the organization for the consultant, an orientation of the consultant to the system/facility, and an expectation for frequent monitoring of the progress of the project. Harris (1995) stresses that the administrator remain involved, as this assures utility of their authority regarding acceptance/implementation of recommendations. Also, administration should continue to monitor for difficulties, screen sensitive content, and be prepared to be a presence with regard to the management and relationship with the consultant.

DILEMMAS REGARDING THE CONSULTANT

Because of the APN's unique role, knowledge and position of influence, the APN has many issues of ethical boundaries and power for which he/she must be responsible and cognizant. Ulshak and Snow-Antle (1990) note the importance of ethical standards. Trust and respect are critical to the utilization of a consultant's recommendations and to the continued use of the consultant. Lippitt and Lippitt (1978) provide a code of ethics for the professional consultant:

1) responsibility for objectivity and integrity;
2) competence to perform the consultation;
3) moral and legal standards;
4) avoidance of misrepresentation;
5) confidentiality;
6) primary consideration for the client's welfare;
7) adherence to professional, rather than economic, standards;

8) integrity in interpersonal relationships;
9) fair remuneration standards;
10) respect for the rights and reputation of the organization; and 11) accurate promotional activities.

Several of these areas warrant special discussion. As one becomes adept in certain areas, it is easy to preconclude and/or apply standardized interventions (Distasio, 1988). The unique contributions of a consultation to a specific situation are jeopardized if this practice occurs without prior client knowledge. Another issue is misrepresentation of expertise or extending one's authority beyond that expertise.

Power is another concern for the consultant. Hersey, Blanchard, and Natemeyer (1979) note that many types of power exist. Van Bree Sneed (1991) notes that the consultant's power is legitimate (power from the position held); referent (based on personality); and expert (based on the possession of special knowledge or skills). Responsible management of this power is accomplished by:

1) respecting the fact that that power places the consultant-client in an unequal relationship;
2) understanding that the consultant's knowledge has a limited scope;
3) resisting the practice of withholding information with the intention of creating dependency;
4) being honest in the presentation of one's abilities and limitations;
5) respecting the aura of influence generated by consultants and avoiding its misuse; and
6) working to assure a balance with regard to the client's perception of that power by providing positive reinforcement to the client.

There are other areas where the consultant must remain vigilant. First, in consultation, one should not push personal opinions, beliefs, values, or biases upon the client. Second, when working in an organization, the consultant must be careful about stressing ideas which conflict with the mission or capabilities of the organization. Third, the parameters of professional/personal conduct should be stressed. Where there are potential differences between client and consultant, resolution or clarification should be sought before the consult proceeds. Fourth, in consultation, the APN must let go of that which has been shared in the consultation There can be a tendency to want to cling to certain turf. Clarity about reasons for retaining certain professional responsibilities, and removing or limiting others, will assist the APN in defining and containing the parameters of the consultation role.

CONCLUSIONS

In summary, consultation can expand the knowledge of nursing and assure a high standard of care by sharing knowledge at multiple levels, with a specific consultee, or with an organization. As the APN consults to a wider and more diverse audience, the specific and ethical responsibilities will assume a greater importance. If theory and practice guide the development of the APN consultant role, the potentials, responsibilities, and opportunities can be ever more challenging to nursing.

REFERENCES

Alvarez, C. (1992). Let's talk about clinical consultation. *Clinical Nurse Specialist, 6,* 117.

Anderson, R. (1985). Alternative revenue sources for nursing departments. *Journal of Nursing Administration,15,* (11), 9–13.

Badger, T. (1988). Mental health consultation with a surgical unit nursing staff. *Clinical Nurse Specialist, 2,* (3), 144–148.

Barron, A. (1989). The CNS as consultant. In A.Hamric & J. Spross (Eds.), *The clinical nurse specialist in theory and practice* (pp. 125–146). Philadelphia: W.B. Saunders.

Benner, P. (1984). *From novice to expert.* Menlo Park, CA: Addison-Wesley.

Beyerman, K. (1988). Consultation roles of the clinical nurse specialist: A case study. *Clinical Nurse Specialist, 2,* (2) 91–95.

Caplan, G. (1970). *The theory and practice of mental health consultation.* New York: Basic Books.

Distasio, C. (1988). Consultative services: guidelines for cost-effective utilization. *Health Care Supervisor, 2,* 1–17.

Edlund, B., Hodges, L., & Poteet, G. (1987). Consultation: Doing it and doing it well. *Clinical Nurse Specialist, 1,* (2) 86–90.

Furlow, L., & Higman, D. (1995). Consultants. When to look outside for help. *Nursing Management, 26,* (5), 49–51.

Harris, M. (1995). Consultants. An administrator's report. *Journal of Nursing Administration, 25,* (7/8), 12–14.

Hersey, P., Blanchard, K., & Natemeyer, W. (1979). Situational leadership, perception, and the impact of power. *Group Organization Studies, 4,* 418–428.

Holt, F. (1984). A theoretical model for clinical specialist practice. *Nursing and Health Care, 5,* 445–449.

Jacobs, C. (1997). Appropriateness guidelines to balance quality and cost. *Hospital Practice, 32*(10), 195–197.

Larsen, J., Risor, O., & Putnam, S. (1997). P-R-A-C-T-I-C-A-L: A step-by-step model for conducting the consultation in a general practice. *Family Practice, 14*(4), 295–301.

Leininger, M. (1988). Leininger's theory of nursing: Cultural care diversity and universality. *Nursing Science Quarterly, 1*(4), 152–160.

Lippitt, G., & Lippitt, R. (1978). *The consulting process in action.* LaJolla, CA: University Associates.

Malone, B. (1989). The CNS in a consultation department. In A. Hamric & T. Spross (Eds.). *The clinical nurse specialist in theory and practice* (pp. 397–413). Philadelphia: Saunders.

Manian, F., & Janssen, D. (1996). Curbside consultation. A closer look at a common practice. *Journal of the American Medical Association, 275*(2), 145–147.

McElhaney, R. & Beare, P. (1998). Expert witness/legal consultant: The importance of data collection. *Clinical Nurse Specialist, 12*(3), 117–120.

McEvoy, M. & Egan, E. (1979). The process of developing a nursing intervention model. *Journal of Nursing Education, 18*(4), 19–25.

Noll, M. (1987). Internal consultation as a framework for clinical nurse specialist practice. *Clinical Nurse Specialist, 1*(1), 46–50.

Norwood, S. (1998a). Making consultation work. *Journal of Nursing Administration, 28*(3), 44–46.

Norwood, S. (1998b). When the CNS needs a consultant. *Clinical Nurse Specialist, 12*(2), 53–58.

ShelleyS. (1994). Interactive consulting: Maximizing your consultant dollar. *Nursing Economics, 12*(5), 272–275.

Ulschak, F., & Snow-Antle, S. (1990). *Consultation skills for health care professionals.* San Francisco: Jossey-Bass.

Van Bree Sneed, N. (1991). Power: Its use and potential for misuse by nurse consultants. *Clinical Nurse Specialist, 5*(1), 58–62.

Chapter 10

RESEARCH

Ruth Lindquist, PhD, RN
Shigeaki Watanuki, RN

> *We are living in a time of unprecedented changes and challenges in our nation's health care system, changes that require nurses to step forward now more than ever and answer the call to advance health through research.*
>
> Patricia A. Grady, PhD, RN

Research is an essential foundation of high-quality care. It is more important that ever to demonstrate the cost-effectiveness of nursing activities in the emerging managed care environment. Innovative approaches to patient care that "make a difference" must be documented. The accumulation of evidence to support the evaluation of the cost-effectiveness of nursing care can be accomplished through nursing research. In fact, nursing's commitment to producing quality, cost-effective patient outcomes requires that a scientific basis for practice be established (Hinshaw, 1989). Substantial strides have been made over the past 25 years

The authors would like to acknowledge the contributions of Keith Hampton, MS, RN, and Mariah Snyder, PhD, RN, FAAN, authors of this chapter in the previous edition.

to increase the amount of nursing research being conducted and to improve the quality of the research. The advent of doctoral education in nursing and the growth in the number of master's-prepared advanced practice nurses (APNs) are two factors having a positive impact on the advancement of nursing research. Nursing truly "came of age" with the institution of the National Center for Nursing Research of the National Institutes of Health in 1985 and the elevation of the Center to Institute status in 1993.

Nursing as a profession is aspiring to build practice on broad and accessible scientific knowledge. Nursing research has become an integral part of the scientific enterprise focused on improving the level of health in the United States (National Center for Nursing Research, 1993). Amidst changes in health care, we as members of the nursing profession need to continue to develop the knowledge that underlies our practice. Many opportunities exist for APNs to expand perspectives and acquire new knowledge for practice.

While studies from other disciplines are helpful, research from the nursing perspective is essential for establishing parameters for using specific interventions in nursing practice and to document the uniqueness of nursing's contribution to the achievement of desired patient outcomes. Research is critical to the development of the discipline of nursing and fundamental to the expansion of the scientific knowledge base underlying nursing practice. However, knowledge accumulated has little value unless it is applied in practice. The accountability of nurses to use new knowledge in practice is clearly described in ANA's standards of Clinical Practice (American Nurses Association, 1991). Research needs to be incorporated into practice to provide high-quality evidence-based care.

Although a discipline cannot expect its clinicians to be expert researchers (Cronenwett, 1995), master's-prepared nurses have unique and critical roles for dissemination and application of research findings to practice settings (Michel & Sneed, 1995). APNs are uniquely prepared and positioned to foster research utilization and to contribute to the conduct of practice-related research. Research is one of the elemental components comprising advanced practice (Benner & Tanner, 1987; Hamric & Spross, 1989), but frequently the one that receives the least attention. A variety of factors may account for the lack of time that APNs devote to research, including lack of administrative support for research, lack of peer support (as few master's-prepared nurses may work in a setting), APNs' responsibility for numerous care units and institutional projects that compete for their time, and the inclusion of few research courses in the APN curriculum (Aiken, 1990). Despite the fact that APNs have indicated that they give minimal attention to research (Stetler & DiMaggio, 1991), the importance of the research component of the APN role cannot be minimized. This chapter will address APNs' involvement in research-based knowledge acquisition, the utilization of research findings in practice, and the APN's role in the research process.

ACQUISITION OF RESEARCH-BASED KNOWLEDGE

Research-based knowledge is the substance required to practice. Recent advances in information technology have reduced the time of information transfer and exponentially expanded the volume of information available to the APN. The rapid expansion of information accessible via the World Wide Web (WWW) provides an enlarged, worldwide resource to be tapped to acquire knowledge and to explore solutions to clinical problems. Electronic mail correspondence and discussion groups such as mailing lists and newsgroups are commonly used communication channels that unite nurses with colleagues on a global scale. Computer technology has expanded the capacity of APNs to access information to stay abreast of new knowledge and to meet the challenges of practice. Competency in the use of computer technology will be vital to a career in nursing in the coming century. It has been observed that:

> new knowledge is generated so rapidly that what health care providers learn during their academic programs is unlikely to be "best practice" within a few years. Professionals cannot plead ignorance of new knowledge. Society demands that health care providers and systems be efficient and effective in helping patients achieve their maximum levels of health. (Cronenwett, 1995, p. 430).

It is common knowledge that all information available is not accurate nor applicable. APNs will need to be prepared to sort, evaluate, and interpret the information available to clients and colleagues. The abilities to read, interpret, and synthesize research are critical to this end. However, it has been estimated that almost half of the practicing nurses have not had a research course (Cronenwett, 1995). Although master's-prepared nurses have been said to have no impact on research utilization (Brett, 1987; Coyle & Sokop, 1990), they were found to be more likely than baccalaureate nurses to relate and to use findings of research in their practice in a more recent study (Michel & Sneed, 1995).

APNs have important roles to play in bringing the findings of research to practice. Continuing education, reading, and professional development will ensure the ongoing increase in the APNs' knowledge and skill to do so. APNs are close to practice and thus can identify clinical problems. They are in key positions to find, interpret and use research findings, and to act as change agents in the practice setting.

Strategies to access research-based information

Many resources and strategies exist to arm nurses with information needed to provide high quality evidence-based practice. Selected key sources and strategies are described.

Comprehensive reviews

Integrative review journals and review articles are rich resources that provide nurses with a summary of the current body of knowledge. Critical and integrative review articles are helpful sources of research information, particularly those that summarize relevant studies and provide overall conclusions from the synthesized findings. These reviews generally provide readers with information on the breadth of the literature reviewed and inform the reader about all relevant studies in the area that was critiqued. Important issues that are unresolved are highlighted (Cooper, 1989). To be useful, reviews need to critique the studies rather than present solely a narrative of the studies. A critique of this nature should be objective in presenting positive and negative aspects of each study. Studies are selected that address the same or similar questions. High-quality reviews of nursing interventions provide an excellent source of information for nurses considering the use of a particular intervention for a specific population. Inclusion of such reviews in clinical nursing journals is beneficial to practitioners.

Clinical focused research journals such as *Applied Nursing Research* and *Clinical Nursing Research* provide useful research-based information that is applicable to clinical practice. Reviews of research related to specific phenomena or areas in nursing are presented in the *Annual Review of Nursing Research* published yearly by Springer Publishing Company (J. Fitzpatrick, 1998). Sigma Theta Tau International's *Online Journal of Knowledge Synthesis for Nursing* is an example of a journal with synthesized knowledge that is available through subscription for online review (Barnsteiner, 1994). Additionally, *The American Journal of Online Journal of Issues in Nursing* is published by Kent State University School of Nursing in partnership with the American Nurses Association.

APNs are encouraged to use review resources for updating clinical practice when relevant, current reviews are available. Other current updated information can be found on the WWW.

Internet and online resources. Some information today is made available only in electronic form (Sparks & Rizzolo, 1998). Knowledge regarding various search engines and databases, including their advantages and disadvantages, as well as strategies of combining these tools, can facilitate APNs to locate WWW resources effectively. Medline, CINAHL (The Cumulative Index to Nursing and Allied Health), and Nursing Collection are bibliographic databases of journal articles. The clinician can combine subjects to narrow the search fields to find desired information. For example, a nurse practitioner may combine a drug name with side effects and specified clinical population and get citations, article abstracts, or full text articles related to side effects of that drug prescribed for the specified population seen in daily practice. Reading "frequently asked questions," trying synonyms for unusual words, and using more than one search tool are strategies that are generally recommended (Sparks & Rizzolo, 1998).

Several useful WWW sites are listed in Table 10.1 with uniform resource locators (URLs). These international, national, or specialty organizations provide research, practice, and funding information at these sites. In addition to those organizations listed, other local organizations may also be useful for research, practice, or grant information including local chapters of Sigma Theta Tau International or specialty nursing organizations, schools of nursing, alumni associations, and state nursing organizations. For more detailed information about the Internet, the reader is referred to a guidebook (Nicoll, 1998).

TABLE 10.1   Selected WWW Sites for Grants and Health-Related Research-based Information

Agency for Health Care Policy and Research <http://www.ahcpr.gov/>
American Academy of Nurse Practitioners <http://www.aanp.org/>
American Association of Critical-Care Nurses <http://www.aacn.org/>
American Association of Neuroscience Nurses <http://www.aann.org/>
American Association of Nurse Anesthetists <http://www.aana.com/>
American College of Nurse-Midwives <http://www.acnm.org/>
American College of Nurse Practitioners <http://www.nurse.org/acnp/>
American Heart Association and Grants Program <http://www.amhrt.org/>
American Nurses Association/American Nurses Foundation
                                        <http://www.nursingworld.org/>
Association of Operating Room Nurses <http://www.aorn.org/>
Emergency Nurses Association <http://www.ena.org/>
Foundations <http://fdncenter.org/>
          Robert Wood Johnson <http://www.rwjf.org/>
          The Pew Charitable Trusts: Health and Human Services
                                        <http://www.pewtrusts.com/>
Midwest Nursing Research Society <http://www.mnrs.org/>
National Institute of Nursing Research <http://www.nih.gov/ninr/>
Oncology Nursing Society <http://www.ons.org/>
Sigma Theta Tau, International <http://www.stti.iupui.edu/>

Synthesis and consensus conferences

Proceedings of conferences sponsored by the National Institutes of Health to review interventions used to treat particular disorders are another source of synthesized research based practice-relevant information. An extensive review of research literature is done by a multidisciplinary panel of experts who are convened to discuss the findings of these studies. At the conclusion of the conference, the experts recommend the most appropriate intervention to use for treating the disorder, and make suggestions for policy and further research. The Midwest Nursing Research Society has sponsored consensus conferences; these are also termed as "synthesis conferences." Nursing experts in a particular area present reviews of relevant studies in the context of these conferences. After discussion by the experts and conference participants, conclusions are drawn regarding the state of the art in the area and the direction that future research should take (Barnfather & Lyon, 1992). The National Institute of Nursing Research has launched online conferences using multimedia technology. Audiences can access conference proceedings from archived streaming video files on the WWW.

The Agency for Health Care Policy and Research (AHCPR) of the United States Public Health Service, Department of Health and Human Services, has facilitated the development of research-based clinical practice guidelines and recommendations to assist clinicians in the prevention, diagnosis, treatment, and management of clinical conditions. Multidisciplinary panels of clinicians and experts are convened to develop statements on patient assessment and management for selected conditions. To accomplish this task, extensive literature searches are completed, as are critical reviews and syntheses. The agency disseminates the research-based practice guidelines to health care providers, policy makers, and the public. Some of the health problems for which guidelines have been developed include acute pain, pressure ulcers, urinary incontinence, cataracts, depression, Alzheimer's Disease, and HIV infection.

APNs can play a pivotal role in assisting health care agencies to change care policies so that research-based AHCPR guidelines are adopted as part of the institutional care policies. In so doing, the organizational practices should be assessed, and any necessary modifications to the guideline should be considered by either a research utilization committee of the organization or a task force for each practice guideline (Kirchhoff & Beck, 1995). Knowledge regarding the individual and the organizational change process is necessary in planning, implementing, and evaluating the practice or care policy changes. APNs have a critical role in the selection, refinement, implementation, and evaluation of the guidelines.

Literature search, review and critique

When comprehensive critical reviews are unavailable or insufficient, literature reviews need to be undertaken. Identifying the studies to be reviewed is time-consuming, but thoughtful attention to the quality and comprehensiveness of the articles reviewed is necessary, especially when developing guidelines or introducing new interventions into practice. Reviews need to include studies that present various perspectives, rather than just including those that support a particular bias or point of view (Moody, 1990). Limiting and focusing the area of interest and the population through careful specification of key search words are crucial steps in the process before identifying the studies to be reviewed. APNs are encouraged to learn skills specific to the electronic search of health and nursing bibliographic databases.

Some study findings in the research literature may be practice-ready, and prescriptions for application are fairly well established. Other research findings are fragmented or not yet synthesized. These require efforts to critique research literature in an area to determine the applicability of the research findings to practice.

Numerous criteria have been developed to guide nurses' efforts to critique research studies to determine their relevance for practice (see Fawcett, 1982, and Killien, 1988). In determining the quality of research reports and the suitability of their findings to practice, numerous factors are considered. These considerations include such things as the appropriateness of the study variables to the practice problem and population to which it will be applied, the quality of the study methods, and the perceived feasibility of the application. The study methods should be clearly described so that the study may be properly evaluated and its merits be assessed. Good clinical judgment should be used to determine if the probability that interventions would be feasible, safe, and effective in the setting to which it is to be transferred. It is advisable that studies are replicated before broadly implementing interventions across practice settings.

Finite research dollars necessitate that the maximum usage be made of studies that have been conducted. Meta-analytic techniques enable more maximal use of research by bringing together the results of a collection of smaller studies into one larger pool of findings for statistical analysis.

Meta-analyses

Meta-analyses go beyond the typical narrative literature review by employing a systematic method of review of experimental studies (Jones, 1994) or descriptive research (Reynolds, Timmerman, Anderson, & Stevenson, 1992). Conducting a meta-analysis of studies related to a particular intervention may provide more information regarding appropriateness, indications, and effectiveness than can be derived from merely looking at the results of the statistical analysis of a large collection of results from selected individual studies (Glass, 1976). Meta-analyses also provide direction for future research (Curlette & Cannella, 1985).

APNs can conduct a meta-analysis when the accumulations of findings that are available in an area are not substantial. Meta-analyses pull together findings of related studies that are identified by specific criteria developed by the author. Meta-analytic techniques are generally employed with very stringent criteria for the inclusion of studies to minimize bias. The criteria for study selection should be decided before examining possible studies for inclusion. Rigor in selecting studies and in conducting the analyses helps to ensure the quality of the meta-analysis. For example, in a meta-analysis of nursing interventions, one scholar selected only studies that had utilized random selection of subjects (Smith, 1988). Meta-analyses can be used to increase the estimates of the effect size (mean differences in standard deviation units) and to increase statistical power. This enables the resolution of uncertainties when results among studies are conflicting or inconclusive, or to answer questions not posed when studies were conducted. A strength of the meta-analytic technique is the ability to arrive at conclusions about interventions even though different instruments were used to measure the outcomes.

Nurse researchers have used meta-analyses to determine outcomes of interventions. For example, a meta-analysis was used to assess efficacy of nonsurgical treatment of chronic pain in returning patients to work (Cutler et al., 1994). In patient education, Theis and Johnson (1995) reported that planned and structured strategies for teaching patients yielded the greatest effect size. In the practices of midwives, Olsen (1997) conducted a meta-analysis of six controlled observational studies of low-risk pregnant women to examine the safety of planned home birth backed up by a hospital system. Planned home birth, as compared with planned hospital birth, was associated with fewer risks and involved fewer medical interventions. Results of meta-analyses can be carefully considered by APNs to determine whether the interventions and practices that have been scrutinized are acceptable and feasible alternatives to existing ones in their practice settings.

Journal clubs

A journal club is a strategy that APNs can implement to increase staff nurses' and their own knowledge about the research process and applicability of findings for practice. Lindquist, Robert, and Treat (1990) noted that journal clubs promote the critique of research in a nonthreatening manner. Their suggestions for a successful journal club included having a regular meeting date, providing an outline to use for critiques, and using a moderator to facilitate discussion. Kirchhoff and Beck (1995) suggested various formats of journal clubs according to the purpose of the club, one article, one journal, or one topic, with/without pre-meeting preparation. Membership of journal clubs varies depending upon the purpose and the organizational climate. For example, if the journal club is aimed at unit-based research utilization, staff nurses and APNs may be included. If it is aimed at bridging the gap between research and practice in a university hospital setting, faculty members and graduate students could be included in addition to the hospital employees. If intended to involve a whole organization, interdisciplinary team members need to be included. If practice changes are desired, scientific merits, risks to the patients, clinical merits, feasibility of implementation, and the potential for clinical evaluation or replication should be considered (Kirchhoff & Beck, 1995).

Conclusions

Caution is a judicious element when applying research findings to practice. From the findings of specific studies, good judgement is needed to determine what is the appropriate population to which results can be generalized. Many interventions require replication studies to further establish the effectiveness or to extrapolate findings from one setting or population to another. Careful clinical evaluation of interventions is warranted so that their suitability for achieving desired outcomes in selected populations may be demonstrated prior to widespread use. Criteria may include such things as strength of research findings of individual studies, overall quality of the research, and amount of evidence (Stetler et al., 1998). Effort should be made to evaluate the application of research findings with respect to clinical practice. "Research utilization" is the term used to describe the process of bringing research findings to practice.

RESEARCH UTILIZATION: SYNTHESIZING AND APPLYING EXISTING KNOWLEDGE IN PRACTICE

Research utilization has been a key concern of nursing professions for more than four decades, yet it has just come of age in the mid-1990s

(Crane, 1995). Research utilization is a crucial process that underlies evidence-based practice, including the updating of organizational policies and clinical procedures and continuous quality improvement in health care. Incorporating research findings into the clinical practice is, however, challenging, because it requires careful critique and "translation" of research findings for application to specific patient populations or practice settings (Tanner, 1987).

Research utilization has been defined as a "systematic process of synthesis, transformation, application, and evaluation of research findings into practice to meet patient care needs" (Lekander, Tracy, & Lindquist, 1994). Two types of utilization, instrumental and conceptual, have been identified (Cronenwett, 1990; Tanner, 1987). Instrumental utilization occurs in a very concrete and direct manner (e.g., specific research findings help clinicians choose a specific action, write a targeted policy, or make a decision). Conceptual utilization is an indirect and cognitive process in that research findings change clinicians' understandings of phenomena or influence the way they think about a given situation. Both types of utilization have value and are used by APNs, but conceptual utilization has a more gradual, almost intangible effect on practice settings and professional over time.

Despite the acknowledged value of research-based practice, nurses have been slow to utilize research findings in practice (Lindquist et al., 1990; Stetler & DiMaggio, 1991; Tanner, 1987). Many nurses have not been taught how to use research methods within the context of their practice. Nursing students in undergraduate and graduate programs have been taught how to conduct research, but not how to utilize research findings. Faculty members, in most cases, have expertise in conducting research, but not in the process of applying the research finding to the practice setting (Crane, 1995). APNs can play a key role in the facilitation of the utilization process.

Some major barriers to research utilization include: (1) availability of research findings; (2) knowledge and attitudes of nurses; and (3) environmental support (Morrola, 1996). The lack of availability of research findings may be attributable to insufficient methods for dissemination and presentation of research findings (Lekander et al., 1994). Research journals may not be readily accessible to clinicians in a small space-constrained practice setting, and research findings found published in clinical and practice journals are limited. The full-text online journals are examples of a solution to this problem.

The lack of research knowledge and negative or indifferent attitudes (a lack of perceived value) of nurses toward research may result from minimal or insufficient educational preparation in research (Funk, Tornquist, & Champagne, 1995; Lekander et al., 1994). Researchers are encouraged to articulate the clinical relevance and specific practice recommendations, because clinicians may be unfamiliar with the language specific to research and statistics.

Environmental barriers include: a lack of authority to change patient care procedures autonomously, a lack of motivation to change practice, funding constraints, and a lack of time due to the multiple role demands on the time of APNs (Carroll et al., 1997; Funk et al., 1995). Administrative support for nurses such as inclusion on a quality improvement committee, provision of expert consultation, or small utilization grants would resolve those environmental barriers.

Research utilization projects and models

Numerous research utilization models are available to assist APNs in the process of systematic application of research to practice. These models vary in their purpose, organizing framework, and target population (individual, group, or institutional) but have similarities in their processes. The process of research utilization models generally includes: identification of clinical problems, assembly and critique of the literature, assessment of applicability of the findings, design of innovation, implementation and evaluation (Nicoll & Beyoa, 1999). APNs as educators can use review articles such as Morrola (1996) and Nicoll and Beyoa (1999) to disseminate research utilization models. The Stetler Model for Research Utilization (Stetler, 1994) has been used in a variety of practical and educational settings to facilitate individual and organizational change process. The model facilitates APNs to make structured decisions appropriately and effectively by way of raising consciousness and ability of critical thinking of potential users. The Iowa Model (Titler et al., 1994) focuses on improvements of the quality of care and has evolved from the Quality Assurance Model Using Research (Watson, Bulechek, & McCloskey, 1987). This model has successfully been used by hospitals and clinics at the University of Iowa and elsewhere.

Other activities

Beyond the role that APNs have in seeking and synthesizing research findings, APNs frequently provide peer review of research manuscripts, abstracts, and research proposals for funding or institutional conduct (Lindquist, Tracy & Treat-Jacobson, 1995). APNs serve as members and chairpersons of nursing research committees, nursing research utilization committees, or research-based policy making bodies. Participating in professional organizations that promote research and the dissemination of research findings are valuable involvements.

When the amount of information available from synthesis of research findings is not sufficient to draw conclusions in the area of interest or concern, APNs may plan or participate in research studies to generate the needed information.

CONDUCTING RESEARCH

Nursing research is essential to develop the knowledge base that may be applied to clinical nursing practice. Although the research of other disciplines may have applicability to practice, nurses may have unique questions, perspectives, methods, and solutions. The "how-to" of research goes beyond the scope of this chapter. For more detailed presentations relating to the conduct of research, the reader is referred to research texts, research colleagues, research seminars, educational offerings, and university graduate coursework.

It is helpful to get expert advice and input from friends, colleagues, and consultants with relevant expertise when embarking on a program of research. A feasibility study with pilot data is a strength, as it can provide empirical data regarding the subjects under investigation as well as evidence to funding agencies of investigator expertise and experience with research subjects and materials. "Pilot work" (a test run) is an advisable first step in the conduct of a research protocol (Lindquist, 1991). Pilot work may provide preliminary data, but it may also be a test ground for methods of recruitment, intervention protocols, and study measures that have been developed or selected.

Many funding sources support the development of a program of research and for ongoing investigations that are built on the strength of insights and knowledge in well-defined areas. Grant awards for research typically increase with the experience of the investigator, paralleling the quality of the proposed research, expertise of the investigative team, and substance of their publications that document excellence. The sizes of the awards are generally larger from regional organizations than from local sources, and larger from national than regional. Local chapters of national and international specialty organizations often award seed monies to support research. Funds may also be solicited from vendors of health-related industries. Research grant information can be found on the WWW and is a timely, up-to-date source of funding availability. Selected examples of organizations with grant programs and their Internet URLs are listed in Table 10.1.

It is advisable to submit a proposal where one judges it will receive the most favorable review. Thus, effort should be given to searching to find the appropriate funding source. The proposal should highlight the potential significance of the outcome relative to the goals of the funding agency to which it is sent. Often, multiple submissions of a grant are required prior to its funding. Many proposals that are not funded are abandoned by the authors even when they contain good ideas.

Often research priorities are developed so that the desired new knowledge relevant to a practice role or specialty area may be systematically developed. The National Center for Nursing Research (NCNR) first formulated a strategic plan for research by developing a National Nursing Research Agenda (Hinshaw, Heinrich, & Bloch, 1989). Research priorities continued to be identified as the NCNR became the National Institute for Nursing Research (NINR) in 1993. Areas of nursing research opportunities for 1999 include clinical interventions for managing symptoms of stroke, respiratory needs of patients: mechanical ventilation, neuroimmunological effects of behavioral interventions, prevention of low birth weight in minority populations, child and adolescent health promotion—reducing and preventing risky behaviors and emerging infection: control through behavioral interventions (National Institute for Nursing Research, 1999). Likewise, priorities have been developed for clinical nursing research by CNSs (Fitzpatrick et al., 1991). Other priorities have been established by practice specialties, including the American Association of Critical-Care Nurses (Lindquist et al., 1993).

Roles

Research expertise, like clinical expertise, is developed and sharpened over time through education and experience. There are many levels of commitment and ways to become involved in the research process. Investigative teams draw together the strengths of individuals who comprise it, and each brings to a project their unique expertise.

The principal investigator takes the overall responsibility for the integrity of the research project. The principal investigator assumes responsibility for writing or coordinating the writing of the proposal and overseeing its conduct. Knowledge about the entire research process is necessary, from proposal generation to analysis, including the dissemination of the study findings. Typically, funding agencies recognize one designated principal investigator who has the overall accountability for the conduct of the project and expenditure of the resources. This person is named first in the list of project investigators. The authority that comes with the accountability of this role may ensure that the project does not become deadlocked in the disagreement among investigators. The principal investigator generally assumes personal as well as professional responsibility for the project's success.

A co-principal investigator shares the leadership in the implementation of a research study. A participant in this role may have been integral to the development of the project and continues an active role through all phases of its conduct and dissemination. A co-investigator or investigator is a member of the research team, but usually assumes responsibility or shares responsibility for a smaller aspect of the study. For example, an APN who is a co-investigator may be responsible for identifying potential subjects for recruitment; implementing an intervention protocol for selected patients; or coordinating other aspects of the study, such as follow-up phone calls or mailings to study participants. The amount of time and degree of responsibility varies from study to study. Regardless of the extent of the involvement, the APNs' experience of being a part of research teams provides opportunities to expand their knowledge about research while contributing to knowledge development.

A project director or study coordinator takes responsibility for the day-to-day conduct of grant activities. Key elements of this role typically include subject recruitment, teaching the necessary protocol activities to staff or data collectors, maintaining protocol integrity as it is implemented, and solving problems that arise throughout the course of the study. APNs are well-suited to the role of project director, since they possess extensive clinical knowledge as well as knowledge of the research process. As project directors, APNs can expand their research expertise and specific knowledge in the area that is under investigation; it is an excellent opportunity for growth for APNs considering a research career.

Collaborator is a general term used to identify individuals working together on a project. The role can carry with it a variety of general or specific responsibilities. For example, an APN in the role of midwife can collaborate on a colleague's project and can assume responsibility for patient recruitment in their clinical work setting. As consultant, APNs may offer their specific expertise to a project. For example, an APN specializing in mental health/psychiatric liaison nursing may be sought to select measures or develop a protocol to identify acute confusion in a study of postoperative falls. A gerontological nurse practitioner may be sought as a consultant to ensure that a study of the effects of early discharge after heart surgery includes age-appropriate measures and protocol accommodations for elderly subjects (e.g., enlarged type font size for enhanced readability; rest periods for elderly subjects if they are fatigued).

Patient outcomes are important research considerations due to the widespread concern regarding the quality of health care (Brooten & Naylor, 1995). APNs in clinical settings are able to identify practice-relevant outcomes and to design research protocols that systematically explore data to meet practice goals. For example, the ambulatory surgical setting provides a cost-effective means of performing surgery. Short-acting anesthetic agents have been developed and used to facilitate more rapid recovery from surgery. However, the relative efficacy of agents for use in particular settings is a significant unresolved issue for nurse anesthetists working in those settings. In one randomized study in the ambulatory setting, discharge time (time from admission to the post anesthesia recovery until discharge home) was examined when patients received general anesthesia with fentanyl versus alfentanil. No differences were found between groups; both agents were judged adequate and comparable for short outpatient procedures (Heather & Martin-Sheridan, 1993).

Challenges and opportunities

Despite the ostensible receptivity of clinicians for studies at clinical sites, there are clinical priorities that may create conflict with respect to study protocol implementation. The conduct of research in service settings is difficult since the immediate clinical physical needs of patients are understandably given higher priority than protocol activities. Attention should be given to design the study protocol to maximize feasibility of protocol adherence in the midst of practice. In the acute care setting, the clinical nurse specialist can play a key role in developing strategies to balance the competing demands of patient care, research, and research utilization (Hickey, 1990; Miller, Johnson, Mackay & Budz, 1997). Research project budgets should be planned so as not to burden staff with protocol activities without remuneration.

Using a personal approach is possibly the most effective method to enlist the cooperation of participating personnel and to engage them in the work (Pollock, 1987). Where there is no sense of ownership by staff involved in protocol implementation, and the top-down approach is used to introduce research into a clinical area, research may be seen as an academic pursuit that is of no relevance to practice. The APN can allay this viewpoint and the derailing of protocols by highlighting the relevance of the research to practice. Where there is no respect between the researcher and the clinician, the clinicians who may be key to recruitment and the success of the protocol may not get involved. An APN who is familiar with the personnel and the work setting can be the spokesperson and assist in integrating the protocol to enhance feasibility. In interactions, the investigator can emphasize the clinical significance of the research, establish an atmosphere of collaboration, and identify informal peer leaders who will support the effort (Parker, Gift, & Creasia, 1989).

Good leadership is a critical ingredient of the APN's role in research. Good communication and the accommodation of the concerns of the practice setting with regards to protocol conduct will facilitate study success. APNs are well positioned to be responsive to the concerns of the researcher and clinicians alike and may play a key role in conflict resolution. APNs may be viewed as clinical "insiders" and, as such, may build interest and relationships in the conduct of research and research utilization among nurses and interdisciplinary professionals. A unit may "take on" a study as a unit project and take pride and ownership in the project.

Research studies conducted at one site are often limited with respect to sample size and generalizability. Multisite research permits increased sample size, broader sampling, faster accrual rates, and more meaningful subgroup analyses through efficient use of resources. Multisite studies also provide for opportunities to learn from other facilities and to expand professional perspectives. However, there are challenges in communication, reliability of measures, standardization of protocol, and data integrity in multisite research. Considerable planning is required to maintain consistency and standardization across divergent practice sites. The APN can serve as the link between sites and investigators and participating personnel in the clinic, hospital or community. For example, Meeropol and Leger (1993) conducted collaborative research through a regional nursing consortium to investigate into the incidence and nature of latex allergies in children. Greater generalizability and more conclusive findings have been brought by the nursing consortium than would be possible in a single practice setting.

Networking is another tool to facilitate multisite research that may be effective for nurse practitioners and primary health providers. Little study has been conducted with regard to the efficacy of primary care providers and the broader applicability of research findings to settings serving the general population. This is partly because of the limited number of subjects in each individual primary care setting (Grey & Walker, 1998). To address this concern, Grey and Walker suggested practice-based research networks for studying clinical problems and practice patterns occurring in community-based primary care practices. The Ambulatory Sentinel Practice Network (ASPN) and Pediatric Research in Office Settings (PROS) are two examples of existing practice-based research networks.

The final stage of the research process is dissemination. Once research findings are generated, they should be made available in summary form with recommendations for their application. Research must be presented to audiences or published so that others can evaluate the work for its clinical utility. It is through dissemination of findings that the information becomes available and may add to the knowledge base. A work that is disseminated in journals, the WWW, and other media becomes accessible to others for the process of research utilization. In the process of dissemination, valuable feedback may also be obtained relative to the application of findings or to future research. Oral and poster presentation skills (Lippman & Ponton, 1989; Ryan, 1989) are frequently developed by APNs. Unfortunately, the findings of many studies have never been presented nor published (Archer Copp, 1990); thus, colleagues have never been informed about findings that may have been potentially relevant to patient care.

CONCLUSION

The ultimate goal of any profession is to establish a base of knowledge that will guide the practice of its members. APNs can and do play an integral role in identifying key practice problems for which research is needed. An equally important role exists for APNs in the utilization of research findings in practice. Although many APNs have not given research a high priority, increased emphasis on this function is needed for the improvement of patient care to occur. The imperative to establish an evidence-based practice as well as an expanding base of clinically relevant research in nursing should be clear. Well-developed programs of research in conjunction with organizational, administrative, and environmental support will foster the climate of openness to innovative practice changes and an evolving evidence-based practice.

The challenges of research utilization and research conduct require leadership from nurses in advanced practice roles. With the exponential growth of information available via new information technologies, APNs are in key positions to sort, synthesize, and interpret information to clients, families, and other professionals. APNs are encouraged to continue their professional development and contribute to quality of evidence-based practice by actively participating in research utilization and in the conduct of research. Involvement in research is essential and provides the avenue and opportunity for continued professional growth and improvement in quality and effectiveness of nursing care.

REFERENCES

Aiken, L. (1990). Charting the future of hospital nursing. *Image: Journal of Nursing Scholarship, 22,* 72–78.

American Nurses Association. (1991). *Standards of clinical nursing practice.* Washington, DC: Author.

Archer Copp, L. (1990). Research dissemination: Bottom line and bottom drawer (editorial). *Journal of Professional Nursing, 6,* 187–188.

Barnfather, J. S. & Lyon, B. L. (1992). *State of the science and implications for nursing theory research and practice.* Indianapolis, IN: Sigma Theta Tau International.

Barnsteiner, J. H. (1994). The online journal of knowledge synthesis for nursing. *Reflections, 20*(2), 10–11.

Benner, P., & Tanner, C. (1987). Clinical judgment: How expert nurses use intuition. *American Journal of Nursing, 87,* 23–31.

Brett, J. K. (1987). Use of nursing practice research findings. *Nursing Research, 36,* 344–348.

Brooten, D., & Naylor, M. (1995). Nurse's effect on changing patient outcomes. *Image: Journal of Nursing Scholarship, 27,* 95–99.

Carroll, D. L., Greenwood, R., Lynch, K. E., Sullivan, J. K., Ready, C. H., &

Fitzmaurice, J. B. (1997). Barriers and facilitators to the utilization of nursing research. *Clinical Nurse Specialist, 11,* 207–212.

Cooper, H. M. (1989). *Integrative research: A guide for literature reviews.* Newbury Park, CA: Sage.

Coyle, L. A., & Sokop, A. G. (1990). Innovation adoption behavior among nurses. *Nursing Research, 39,* 176–180.

Crane, J. (1995). The future of research utilization. *Nursing Clinics of North America, 30,* 565–577.

Cronenwett, L. R. (1990). Improving practice through research utilization. In S. Funk, E. Tornquist, M. Champagne, L. Copp, & R. Wiese (Eds.), *Key aspects of recovery: Improving nutrition, rest, and mobility* (pp. 7–22). New York: Springer Publishing Company.

Cronenwett, L. R. (1995). Effective methods for disseminating research findings to nurses in practice. *Nursing Clinics of North America, 30,* 429–438.

Curlette, W. L., & Cannella, K. S. (1985). Going beyond the narrative summarization of research findings: The meta-analysis approach. *Research in Nursing and Health, 8,* 293–301.

Cutler, R. B., Fishbain, D. A., Rosomoff, H. L., Abdel-Moty, E., Khalil, T. M., & Rosomoff, R. S. (1994). Does nonsurgical pain center treatment of chronic pain return patients to work? A review and meta-analysis of the literature. *Spine, 19,* 643–652.

Fawcett, J. (1982). Utilization of nursing research findings. *Image: Journal of Nursing Scholarship, 14,* 57–59.

Fitzpatrick, E., Sullivan, J., Smith, A., Mucowski, D., Hoffmann, E., Dunn, P., Trice, M., & Grosso L. (1991). Clinical nursing research priorities: A Delphi study. *Clinical Nurse Specialist, 5,* 94–99.

Fitzpatrick, J. (Ed.) (1998). *Annual review of nursing research.* New York: Springer Publishing Company.

Funk, S. G., Tornquist, E. M., & Champagne, M. T. (1995). Barriers and facilitators of research utilization: An integrative review. *Nursing Clinics of North America, 39,* 395–407.

Glass, G. V. (1976). Primary, secondary, and meta-analysis of research. *Educational Researcher, 5,* 3–8.

Grady, P. A. (1996). The key to excellence in nursing practice. *Cardiovascular Nursing, CVN Fall Newsletter,* 5–8.

Grey, M., & Walker, P. H. (1998). Practice-based research networks for nursing. *Nursing Outlook, 46,* 125–129.

Hamric, A. B., & Spross, J. A. (1989). *The clinical nurse specialist in theory and practice.* New York: Grune & Stratton.

Heather, D. J., & Martin-Sheridan. D. (1993). Discharge time in patients who receive fentanyl or alfentanil for general anesthesia. *Nurse Anesthesia, 4,* 160–165.

Hickey, M. (1990). The role of the clinical nurse specialist in the research utilization process. *Clinical Nurse Specialist, 4,* 93–96.

Hinshaw, A. S. (1989). Nursing science: The challenge to develop knowledge. *Nursing Science Quarterly, 2,* 162–171.

Hinshaw, A. S., Heinrich, J., & Bloch, D. (1989). Evolving clinical nursing research priorities: A national endeavor. *Journal of Professional Nursing, 4,* 398, 458–459.

Jones, A. (1994). An introduction to meta-analysis. *Respiratory Care, 39,* 34–49.

Killien, M. G. (1988). Disseminating and using research findings. In N. Woods & M. Catanzaro (Eds.), *Nursing research: Theory and practice.* (pp. 479–497). St. Louis: C.V. Mosby.

Kirchhoff, K. T., & Beck, S. L. (1995). Using the journal club as a component of the research utilization process. *Heart & Lung: Journal of Critical Care, 24,* 246–250.

Lekander, B. J., Tracy, M. F., & Lindquist, R. (1994). Overcoming obstacles to research utilization in critical care. *AACN Clinical Issues in Critical Care Nursing, 5,* 115–123.

Lindquist, R. (1991). Don't forget the pilot work! *Heart & Lung, 20,* 91–92.

Lindquist, R., Banasik, J., Barnsteiner, J., Beecroft, P. C., Prevost, S., Riegel, B., Sechrist, K., Strzelecki, C., & Titler, M. (1993). Determining AACN's research priorities for the 90s. *American Journal of Critical Care, 2,* 110–117.

Lindquist, R., Robert, R. C., & Treat, D. (1990) A clinical practice journal club: Bridging the gap between research and practice. *Focus on Critical Care, 17,* 402–406.

Lindquist, R., Tracy, M. F., & Treat-Jacobson, D. J. (1995). Peer review of nursing research proposals. *American Journal of Critical Care, 4,* 59–65.

Lippman, D. T., & Ponton, K. G. (1989). Designing a research poster with impact. *Western Journal of Nursing Research, 11,* 477–485.

Meeropol, E., & Leger, R. R. (1993). Latex allergy: Collaborative nursing research using a consortium model. *Clinical Nurse Specialist, 7,* 254–257.

Michel, Y., & Sneed, N. V. (1995). Dissemination and use of research findings in nursing practice. *Journal of Professional Nursing, 11,* 306–311.

Miller, C., Johnson, J. L., Mackay, M., & Budz, B. (1997). The challenges of clinical nursing research: Strategies for successful conduct. *Clinical Nurse Specialist, 11,* 213–216.

Moody, L. E. (1990). Meta-analysis: Qualitative and quantitative methods. In L. E. Moody (Ed.), *Advancing nursing science through research* (Vol. 2, pp. 70–110). Newbury Park, CA: Sage.

Morrola, C. A. (1996). Research utilization and the continuing/staff development educator. *Journal of Continuing Education in Nursing, 27,* 168–175, 192.

National Center for Nursing Research. (1993). *Developing knowledge for practice: Challenges and opportunities.* Bethesda, MD: Author.

National Institute for Nursing Research. (1999). 1999 NINR Areas of Research Opportunity. Available on-line: http://www.nih.gov/ninr/1999AoRO.htm.

Nicoll, L. H. (1998). Nurses' guide to the Internet (2nd ed.). Philadelphia: Lippincott-Raven.

Nicoll, L. H. & Beyoa, S. C. (1999). Research utilization. In J. A. Fain (Ed.).

Reading, understanding, and applying nursing research: A text and workbook (pp. 261–280). Philadelphia: F. A. Davis.

Olsen, O. (1997). Meta-analysis of the safety of home birth. *Birth: Issues in Perinatal Care & Education, 24,* 4–16.

Parker, B. J., Gift, A. G., & Creasia, J. L. (1989). Clinical research with patients in crisis: Pitfalls and solutions. *Clinical Nurse Specialist, 3,* 178–181.Pollock, S. E. (1987). Clinical nursing research: The needed link for unifying professional nursing. *Clinical Nurse Specialist, 1,* 8–12.

Reynolds, N. R., Timmerman, G., Anderson, J., & Stevenson, J. S. (1992). Meta-analysis for descriptive research. *Research in Nursing & Health, 15,* 467–475.

Ryan, N. M. (1989). Developing and presenting a research poster. *Applied Nursing Research, 2,* 52–55.

Smith, M. C. (1988). *Meta-analysis of nursing intervention research.* Birmingham, AL: University of Alabama-Birmingham.

Sparks, S. M., & Rizzolo, M. A. (1998). World Wide Web search tools. *Image: Journal of Nursing Scholarship, 30,* 167–171.

Stetler, C. B. (1994). Refinement of the Stetler/Marram model for application of research findings to practice. *Nursing Outlook, 42,* 15–25.

Stetler, C. B., Brunell, M., Giuliano, K. K., Morsi, D., Prince, L., & Newell-Stokes, V. (1998). Evidence-based practice and the role of nursing leadership. *Journal of Nursing Administration, 28*(7/8), 45–53.

Stetler, C. B., & DiMaggio, G. (1991). Research utilization among clinical nurse specialists. *Clinical Nurse Specialist, 5,* 151–155.

Tanner, C. A. (1987). Evaluating research for use in practice: Guidelines for the clinician. *Heart and Lung, 16,* 424–431.

Theis, S. L., & Johnson, J. H. (1995). Strategies for teaching patients: A meta-analysis. *Clinical Nurse Specialist, 9,* 100–120.

Titler, M. G., Kleiber, C., Steelman, V., Goode, C., Takel, B., Barry-Walker, J., Small, S., & Buckwalter, K. (1994). Infusing research into practice to promote quality care. *Nursing Research, 43,* 307–313.

Watson, C. A., Bulechek, G. M., & McCloskey, J. C. (1987). QAMUR: A quality assurance model using research. *Journal of Nursing Quality Assurance, 2,* 21–27.

Chapter **11**

THE ADVANCED PRACTICE NURSE AS A CHANGE AGENT

Helen E. Hansen, PhD, RN, CNAA

For 45 years clinical nurse specialists, nurse practitioners, nurse-midwives, and nurse anesthetists have functioned as agents of change in health care. Advanced practice nurses (APNs) have introduced sophisticated new interventions for meeting the unique needs of diverse populations. In a variety of settings, APNs have initiated innovations in technology, patient education, coordination, and continuity of health care transitions, and they have exercised expert clinical, staff development, and consultative skills. The role of APNs as change agents also has extended to care delivery innovations, such as primary nursing, case management, development and application of critical pathways, and creating programs to improve health and maintain wellness in a highly managed care environment. In addition, APNs have functioned as driving forces in focusing research efforts on important clinical problems. Change agent activity by APNs has ranged from addressing the unique problems of individual clients and their families to disentangling the dysfunctions and inefficiencies of service processes within and between health care agencies. Irrespective of the range of change activities, the primary purpose of APN involvement in change is to improve the quality of and access to clinical care for clients and their families, particularly for those whose health status is precarious.

In rural New Hampshire, two nurse-midwives, one of whom is a family nurse practitioner, provide basic health care for 4,300 people (Freudenheim, 1997). They are reimbursed the same amount as physicians providing the same care. Several health maintenance organizations in New York City pay a group of nurse practitioners $50 to $60 for each primary care patient visit, the same amount as primary care physicians are reimbursed (Miller, 1998). Despite considerable opposition from the medical establishment, APNs, often in collaboration with schools of nursing, in some cases supported by foundations, have been breaking new ground in the national effort to assure access to quality care that is patient- and community-oriented.

Given this history of involvement in change, APNs will continue to assume change agent roles. Creative change agency is needed as health care reform faces an uncertain future in terms of improving access, assuring positive client outcomes, and preventing costs from rising. Fagin and Schwartz (1993) suggested that independent APNs become primary care gatekeepers in a reorganized health care system that focuses on promotion and prevention and reduction of the need for expensive high technology. In this role, APNs perform a triage function for health care networks and independently make decisions about what providers and services patients use. While this approach is debated hotly, especially with physicians, Fagin's suggestion effectively matches the nation's needs for managing health care services and is based on research findings that clearly indicate that the skills and knowledge of APNs are well suited to providing quality, cost-effective primary care (Office of Technology Assessment, 1986; Safriet, 1992).

According to Gibson, Ivancevich, and Donnelly (1982), change agents, because of their unique expertise, information or knowledge, relationships, and often their position in the organization, provide unique perspectives on complex situations and can challenge the status quo. Change agents may anticipate the need for change, initiate change, or shape and support change that is underway. They participate in any or all aspects of the diagnostic, planning, implementation, and evaluation stages of the change process. APNs are positioned and skilled to influence many aspects of clinical, organizational, and policy change.

APNs function as change agents either intentionally or opportunistically. As agents of intentional or planned change, they use deliberative processes to precipitate and foster change. This approach, often referred to as planned change, has been described extensively in the literature and is outlined in Table 11.1.

As opportunistic change agents, APNs affect individual and organization-

TABLE 11.1 Intentional or Planned Change Process

Engagement Phase: Establish Trust and Credibility

Designate target change setting.
Establish necessary political, working, and interpersonal relationships with groups and individuals. Secure resources.

ProblemlOpportunity Phase: Create a Vision

Identify opportunity for change.
Clarify the change opportunity. Analyze objective and subjective data related to the problem.
Specify change outcomes.
Win involvement and consensus of key stakeholders.
Generate, explore, test, select strategies.
Write a change proposal.
Gain commitment and approval of proposal.

Implementation Phase: Transformation

Create a step-by-step implementation plan, including what will be done, by whom, and when. Designate an implementation team.
Develop contingency plans for capitalizing on driving forces and overcoming restraining forces.
Lead or support the implementation team. Facilitate periodic assessments of the change process. Monitor the reception and integration of change.
Champion the change formally and informally.

al performance by noticing (when others do not) an opportunity for improvement in structure, process, or outcome in the service setting. Largely through the thoughtful use of personal power (expert, informational, referent, connection), political influence, and a tactical presence in the clinical situation, APNs effect subtle, incremental changes in the behavior of others. Through either intentional or opportunistic means, change agents, by definition, also can stimulate change in the functioning of a system. Observation of clinical practices that deviate substantially from the "best practice frontier" (Finkler & Wirtschafter, 1993) is one way that APNs identify change opportunities. The principles for effecting change, either intentionally or opportunistically, are the same in terms of (a) selecting and focusing on change opportunities with potential to yield significant benefits, (b) building and maintaining political and interpersonal relationships needed to engage others in change efforts, (c) expertly planning and guiding the change activity or several change activities simultaneously, and (d) continuously monitoring the change process, giving and receiving feedback, and helping others make adjustments.

APNs are often especially effective change agents because of their boundary-spanning and horizontal-linkage roles in most organizations and in the community. They regularly span boundaries as they communicate with agencies and individuals outside the clinical setting in their efforts to secure resources for clients. According to Daft (1986), individuals who span boundaries detect and process changes in the external environment, such as in the community, with other health providers, consumers, and their families, and they represent the organization to the external environment. Through boundary-spanning, APNs often detect the need for change before others, and they send information to the internal environment that may maximize the organization's opportunity to be first in responding to emerging needs.

In horizontal linkage roles, APNs continually share information and ideas across professional disciplines, departments, service areas, and specialties. They facilitate joint problem analysis, problem-solving, and new program and service development. Both boundary-spanning and horizontal linkages are essential to the change process in clinical practice and organizations. Boundary-spanning is necessary to permit detection of needs and opportunities for change and to maintain a reality-oriented connection with active and potential clients. Horizontal linkages are necessary for organizational mobilization and coordination in the face of identified opportunities and needs for change. The APN is also often in the position to recognize how the community is "client" and to interpret for the organization or health agency changes in the community's health status and needs and propose solutions. Ervin and Young (1996) provided an example of how a nursing center in a low-income, underserved community in Chicago was developed based on principles of boundary-spanning, which included colleges of nursing, medicine, and pharmacy, a community council, and a Head Start program. The innovative program, led by APNs, significantly improved immunization rates among young children, reduced the rate of low-birthweight deliveries, improved prenatal care seeking in the first trimester, and generally improved the accessibility and acceptability of care in the community.

OPPORTUNITIES TO INFLUENCE CHANGE

APNs traditionally have initiated change specific to some aspect of caring for patients in a single setting. A clinical nurse specialist or nurse practitioner typically tackles problems and opportunities for introducing new health interventions in a relatively circumscribed situation with a limited number of clients. Examples of this kind of change include Noone's (1987) introduction of a new critical care flowsheet in the intensive and coronary care units and Walsh's (1989) report of the establishment of a hospital-wide wound care program. Opportunities of this kind will continue to offer APNs challenges for initiating change. They will remain important because analysis of clinical conditions and the need for innovation begins at the case level. The stimulus for research and intervention often comes from individual clinical experience.

More recently, APNs have become involved in the health of broader populations of patients, families, and communities. Naylor and Brooten (1993), for example, described the effects of clinical nurse specialist practice on outcomes of low-birthweight infants, children with chronic illnesses, acutely ill adults, and the hospitalized elderly. Research on clinical nurse specialist functions and models of clinical nurse specialist practice showed that advanced practice nursing has a significant effect on patient outcomes and the cost and quality of care. Aiken et al. (1993) found that nurse practitioners generated outcomes comparable to those of MDs in a small sample of HIV-infected patients. The investigators concluded that nurse practitioners could improve access to care for patients with HIV-related illness. Keane and Richmond (1993), in proposing the role of tertiary care nurse practitioner, suggested that nurse practitioners could improve the ability of acute care facilities to meet the increasing needs for quantity and intensity of care in the face of downsized residency programs, increasing numbers of medically vulnerable groups, and rising health care costs. Bissing, Alfred, Afford, and Bellig (1997) reported that the quality outcomes for two matched groups of neonates, one group cared for by medical house staff and the other by neonatal nurse practitioners (NNPs), were comparable. In addition, they found that the cost of care for the infants cared for by the NNPs was, on average, $18,240 less per infant than the cost for infants cared for by medical house staff. These studies indicate that the scope of advanced practice change agency is shifting from an individual focus to a population and systems focus. It also suggests that APNs improve dramatically the care of underserved vulnerable populations in a cost-effective manner. Given that millions of children and vulnerable adults remain un-and underinsured, despite the managed care movement and welfare reform, APNs are more and more likely to assume leadership roles as primary providers in the 21st century.

APNs are positioned to create change in the delivery of services to intensely and chronically ill, underserved, or vulnerable populations because of their boundary-spanning and horizontal linkage roles within health care organizations and across systems. Individuals in boundary-spanning and horizontal-linkage roles possess unique perspectives on the activities of institutions. For example, APNs are positioned to observe the efficiency with which services are provided to clients during a clinic visit. Problems, delays, errors in registration, completion of diagnostic procedures, timeliness of reports, responsiveness of consultants, availability of equipment, supplies, and appliances promptly come to the attention of APNs. APNs coordinate multiple services and organize and interpret patient information from a variety of sources. Often they identify psychosocial or cultural barriers that prevent individuals from seeking care or following through with treatment. In boundary spanning and horizontal linkages, APNs often must resolve conflicts among professional staff related to communication, differences in priorities, and client frustration with systems inefficiency and ineffectiveness. Making an impact as a change agent in these circumstances is most challenging and requires role flexibility, selecting targets for change, using thoughtful collaboration strategies, and a broad range of technical, administrative, and interpersonal skills. APNs have the unprecedented opportunity to influence the transformation of health care in partnership with administrators, clinical staff, other disciplines, and suppliers of technology and pharmaceuticals.

Opportunities for change agency by APNs are increasing because today's health care organizations and agencies are faced with both environmental and internal forces for change. Environmental forces can be classified as (a) economic or marketplace forces, (b) technology, and (c) social and political pressures (Gibson et al., 1982). Rapidly escalating costs (including those associated with advances in clinical and managerial technology), health care reform, consumer dissatisfaction and insecurity about health care coverage, and lack of access represent growing pressures on health care providers.

Internal pressures come from behavioral and process sources. They include

(a) the drive for increased efficiency, effectiveness, and productivity;
(b) a leaner, more diverse, less stable workforce;
(c) competition and confusion among professionals over roles in primary care and case management;
(d) the requirement for competency-based training and development of staff;
(e) discontent and anxiety among professional staff;
(f) the demand for analysis and revision of work processes;

(g) quality initiatives; and
(h) the need to improve coordination and collaboration among the members of the multidisciplinary team.

Change in health care systems also faces strong forces of resistance. Economic stakes are high. Health care organizations and agencies remain bureaucratic and hierarchical, which makes it difficult to plan flexibly for the future. Dominant players, such as physicians, traditionally make decisions outside of the collaborative decision making structure of the organization and many continue to resist the need to work in concert with institutional decision makers. Professional staff perceive threats from change and become insecure about their roles and jobs. They often lack the skills, tools, and time needed to effectively analyze and correct dysfunctional work processes or to plan creatively for new roles. APNs can view these forces as conditions calling for their unique problem-solving abilities.

In addition to change agent activity related to external and internal forces for change, APNs have opportunities to become involved in activities associated with national health priorities. Children's health is a prominent concern. Immunization, safety, and effects of violence, abuse, drugs, and alcohol are receiving national attention and increasing support in terms of public programming and research funding. Women's health in general, and the needs of aging women especially, are receiving more research attention. More pressure is being placed on the federal government to improve funding for cancer research, especially in the areas of prevention and early detection. A heightened awareness of the role APNs can play in attending to preventive health care needs and in minimizing the use of intrusive, expensive, and unnecessary technology is emerging. APNs are well prepared to participate in research activities that serve to identify and test interventions designed to deal with critical health issues that have been identified as national priorities through initiatives such as *Healthy People 2010*. Change agents in the health care environment have unique opportunities to provide leadership in shaping health care delivery in the future so that national priorities are addressed. APNs, who understand both the clinical and administrative challenges in their practice settings, occupy an excellent position for facilitating the change process through a variety of means. APNs are also uniquely positioned to build on the important relationships with physicians and other professionals in maintaining a productive work situation, a welcoming service environment, engaging in community outreach, and negotiating with payers for health care.

MODELS

Various models may serve as frameworks for the APN change agent. Some are more traditional and familiar than others. Some models require new perspectives on change and change agency.

The usefulness of any given model depends on the nature of change in the APN's setting and beliefs about change. Inherent in the evolution of APN change agent functions is role ambiguity, overlap, and conflict. Hamric and Taylor (1989) suggested that the role development of clinical nurse specialists in hospitals experiencing major change is in a "reorganization" phase. Most agencies undergoing major change engage in an evaluation of APN roles. Some of the questions about the role and value of APNs are quite familiar. They include: What are the financial contributions of APNs to the institution? What are the proper volume and types of services they should supply? How does graduate education affect the relevance of advanced practice nursing? What are the appropriate reporting and working relationships of APNs, especially vis-à-vis physicians and non-nurse administrators? How does the organization justify the salary costs and number of APN full-time equivalents? What kinds of new APN roles are indicated by reforms in the health care system (e.g., emergency services, women's health, tertiary care nurse practitioners; pediatric rheumatology clinical nurse specialist; combined practitioner/clinical specialist roles)? To what extent should APNs extend the availability of medical services, as opposed to expanding the scope of nursing care?

On the other hand, some questions about advanced practice nursing are new. To what extent will APNs compete with physicians for the primary gatekeeper role in health care systems? How can APNs improve the ability of the health care system to provide greater access to underserved populations at lower costs? What role can APNs play in improving health promotion and disease prevention? How will APN practice affect the educational preparation of primary medical practitioners? What role can APNs play in maximizing the benefits of managed care, remedying serious shortcomings, or creating alternatives? APNs, administrators, and physicians who work with them, regardless of the setting, confront these questions regularly. Some of these confrontations are highly productive and satisfying, while others are unproductive and frustrating. Wrestling with these issues is inevitable as health care change, and APNs seek to shape its future.

APNs recognize that, as health care services come under increasing pressure related to cost and quality, they must reexamine how they meet the needs of clients in light of the entire system's (providers, payers, employers) growing emphasis on scrupulously managing resources. APNs are experienced in negotiating, formally or informally, with employing agencies about the services they will provide. Astute APNs view these ongoing negotiations and renegotiations as opportunities to better tie their unique portfolio of skills to the changing needs of the agency and the public and to continuously refine the responses to the questions posed above. The questions related to advanced nursing practice and health care organizations present opportunities for change that may be guided by the APN. Several models may be considered in conceptualizing and orienting the APN's approach to change in a given setting. APNs must assess the nature of change in their organizations, agencies, or communities in order to plan and implement successful change strategies.

Kaluzny and Hernandez (1988) describe three models of organizational change: rational, resource dependency, and organizational ecology. These may be useful in considering how APNs may view change dynamics in their settings and design strategies for the future. The rational model is focused primarily on internal aspects of the organization. Change is viewed as a linear process involving four basic stages: recognition of the need for change, identification of a course of corrective action, implementation of a plan, and institutionalization of the change. Most of the traditional models of change (e.g., Havelock, 1973; Lewin, 1958; Lippitt, 1973) reflect a rational approach to change. Welch (1990) provides an excellent comparison of the three models. The direction of change—in behaviors, structures, or an integration of behaviors and structures—is determined by goals, objectives, action plans, programs, and activities. Change is generally short-term and timebound.

The resource dependency model focuses on the relationship between the organization and the environment in terms of the mutual interdependency of the two. Interdependency results from the organization's need for resources from the environment and the environment's need for services. Change involves assessment of environmental factors and appropriate responses on the part of the organization. The time frame for change is intermediate and ongoing.

The organizational ecology model views change from a broad "evolutionary natural-selection" perspective (Kaluzny & Hernandez, 1988, p. 402). Change is not so much directional as simply unfolding. The ecology model emphasizes concepts of life-cycle growth and decline, uncertainty, variation, and reforming structures. Change is not timebound and is relatively unpredictable.

Wheatley (1992) suggests a fourth model, somewhat similar to the organizational ecology model. She proposes that organizations are necessarily in disequilibrium internally and in relation to the environment, and that disequilibrium is necessary to the organization's growth, change, and renewal. In Wheatley's view, organizations appear to be in chaos. However, within the disorder and chaos reside activities that reflect underlying orderly, purposeful change. Close observation reveals movement indicating self-organization and self-renewal. Change is continual and patterned.

Both the ecology model and the "chaos" models are useful in understanding today's health care environment. Although organizations continue to employ time-honored strategic planning methods to "rationally" prepare and position for the future, the internal instability of the organization and the unpredictability of the external environment limit the effectiveness of traditional planning for change. Traditional planning must continue to occur, but Kaluzny and Hernandez (1988) and Wheatley (1992) suggest that alternative, more flexible perspectives on change in organizations be adopted.

The APN should become skillful in assessing change in the work setting objectively, from an emotional and social distance. APNs should observe and analyze the organization and key players' relationships to their internal and external environments (interdependent, interactive, independent, insular); how the organization responds to internal and external pressures for change (proactively, reciprocally, reactively, aggressively, resistively); how the organization views change (as learning opportunity, challenge, nuisance, threat); what the organization values as outcomes of change (improved positioning, equilibrium, stability, security); what change looks and feels like as it's occurring (patterned transitions in growth, steps and stages, lurching and stumbling, chaos and confusion, panic).

To such an analysis of change dynamics one can apply one of the change models in order to formulate an understanding of and framework for the change experience in the setting, and to select strategies that effectively facilitate change. For example, if the organization's relationship to change is highly rational and linear, precisely orchestrated planning strategies may be successfully employed. The APN will need to learn how to use and participate in strategic planning activities. If the organization experiences change as unpredictable and troublesome, its key members will seek to anticipate short-term effects of isolated external factors and make the minimally necessary tactical maneuvers to avoid adverse consequences. In this situation, the APN will seek to become adept at detecting risks and threats and troubleshooting procedures and communications. If the organization relates to change as inherently necessary, and views stability and security as unlikely or undesirable, then the APN will want to look for underlying consistent patterns of response to change that are not necessarily formally or explicitly sanctioned. Individuals or groups may be formed to tackle a problem or generate an innovation to respond to an opportunity. In this situation, the APN may want to gain a good understanding of the relationships and processes generally employed when change is initiated, and look for and create opportunities to participate in and ultimately lead change activity.

In order to become effective change agents, APNs must become familiar and comfortable with the change style of the setting and its key players. Then they must develop the role(s) and requisite skills that are most valued and needed for leadership in the change process. After APNs have become familiar with and adept at facilitating change in terms of the existing change paradigm, they may then wish to introduce new strategies based on different models.

CHANGE AGENT ROLES

APNs may exercise change agency from any of the traditional dimensions of the role: clinician/practitioner, consultant, educator, researcher. Typically, change agency associated with these dimensions has focused on patient care units or caseloads of patients unique to a specific specialty, discipline, disease, or diagnosis. More recently, the APN's focus has broadened significantly to include entire populations of clients and their families. Direct advanced nursing practice is occurring more routinely within interdisciplinary teams accountable for the management of populations of clients. The care of client populations has been organized into service or product lines that cover entire episodes of health care. Service lines are more fluid and flexible than the highly compartmentalized, procedure-bound, individually delivered diagnostic and therapeutic procedures of the past. Some patients' total care needs (e.g., those in pain or with HIV infection) span across service lines, and new systems of care provide for the coordination of their care regardless of focus of the immediate need. APNs have always maintained a broad scope of practice not limited to a single hospitalization or outpatient visit. The movement to service or product line care delivery is very compatible with the APN's capabilities as clinician/practitioner, consultant, educator, or researcher.

Some key differences exist in advanced practice nursing's traditional roles in today's rapidly changing health care system. The focus of change influence must shift to the population rather than the geographically defined group. APNs must think in terms of innovations in interventions that will impact both the quality and cost of care delivered to the cohorts or communications of clients and the families. APNs must think of change agency in terms of the interdisciplinary team and the organization, as well as the individual.

For instance, an adult nurse practitioner in the employ of a group of cardiologists collaborates with inpatient nursing staff to plan and coordinate the development of intensive clinic-based follow-up services for congestive heart failure patients. Both groups of nurses, along with discharge planners, patient educators, the utilization review coordinator, and the social worker, recognize that, due to very short lengths of stay, the educational and needs of these frail elders and their family caregivers are complex and ongoing. For them to remain at home and in a stable physiological and psychosocial state requires ongoing support and modification of treatment. A follow-up program will help prevent unnecessary and untimely rehospitalization.

In clinical, consultation, educational, and research activities, the APN should consider how a team, task force, or interest group could work together to improve the quality of care. Teams may work on assuring the appropriate use of technology, enhancing systems of communication and care management, raising the efficiency of care activities, better satisfying clients, and adding to the knowledge base for practice. All change must be thought of as requiring the involvement of others. Through the traditional roles of clinician, consultant, and educator, the APN should encourage the team to experiment and pilot test new methods. Change should be viewed not so much as shifting from one method to another, but rather as an evolutionary, continuous, developmental process. APNs should be expert at helping teams devise innovations that reference the mission of the organization, address significant needs, secure commitment, and serve as the foundation for the next innovation.

In some cases, as consultants, the APNs will provide internal organizational development advice. According to McDougall (1987), the consultation role must become broader. It should not remain limited to clinical interventions, but address organizational strengths and weaknesses, structural or behavioral processes, work flow, interpersonal relations, communications, and intra- and intergroup relations. This expanded dimension is appropriate because APNs hold unique positions in observing and assessing both the system of care and clients' needs.

Finally, increasingly APNs should recognize the importance of research, research utilization, and evidence-based practice as valuable instruments of change. As the base of clinical research grows, APNs have access to an expanding knowledge base for clinical innovation. The APN must remain current in terms of the research knowledge base and continually seek to identify opportunities to apply new findings to specific clinical conditions as well as to care delivery processes. Applications include standards, nursing care delivery models, interdisciplinary collaboration, case management and critical pathways, and patient support systems. As the knowledge base related to persons' health experiences increases, APNs, serving as client advocates, can provide leadership and guidance to the health care team in redesigning care delivery.

APNs may assume new roles as change agents in health care in the future. Examples of new roles include nurse manager partner; outcomes manager; program, project, service line, or product line manager; physician partner; and/or systems analyst. Each role requires the acquisition of skills and knowledge not traditionally associated with advanced practice, but that are well within the grasp of APNs who recognize the organizational scope of their roles. All of the new roles assume that APNs will take an active part in redesigning health services and will assume greater accountability for population-focused client outcomes.

In inpatient settings, APNs may form formal partnerships with nurse managers or administrators, as suggested by Ponte, Higgins, James, Fay, and Madden (1993). In conjunction with nurse managers, APNs may assume accountability for patient cost and quality outcomes. They will create and implement case management strategies for high-volume and high-risk patient populations and will formulate strategies for addressing variances in nursing practice. APNs will initiate projects in collaboration with nurse managers to improve care management supported by research and staff development. APNs will also routinely initiate programs and projects to carry out innovations and improvements within the nursing service and health care agency. As outcomes manager, in any setting, APNs will create and oversee case management strategies. APNs will facilitate the development of critical pathways and other tools for use by the entire interdisciplinary team for managing the care of patients over extended health care experiences. They will lead to the creation of monitoring, documentation, and tracking systems that facilitate their work and that of others. APNs will develop communication patterns and systems that facilitate the coordination of clients' care through multiple, complex transitions related to phases of illness and wellness, across settings, and through the life span. In this role, APNs will make major contributions to outcomes research and effective systems, as well as clinical interventions. In terms of case management, APNs will help to shape the case management role(s), systems, and tools of the future. They will bring real sophistication and scope to the function of case management and the systems of case management that health networks will employ to ensure quality outcomes, cost control, and equitable access. In addition, APNs will promote case and care management strategies that satisfy client needs for coordination, communication, and integration of care.

Increasingly, APNs will exercise their leadership skills in creating and managing new programs, projects, services, and product lines. Because APNs often identify opportunities to improve services, they are called upon to design the programs and manage the projects that will generate significant change.

Project management involves the exercise of organizational leadership to create a new health product, often a new program or service. The APN may facilitate the work of multiple specialists from several vertically organized departments to develop a new service, which will then be managed by the APN or some other manager. As Hermann, Alexander, and Kiely (1992) point out, project management is a change strategy because it employs planning methods to change targeted aspects of an organization's mission and operations. In the project management role, the APN must recognize the need and importance of the desired change, select the specialists who will participate in designing the change, and then lead this diverse group through a compressed planning process. Once the project has been completed, the APN may assume responsibility for managing the resulting program, service, or product line on an ongoing basis. Program, service, or product line management usually involves management and continuous improvement of a package of activities and services that aim to deal with a specific health care concern, e.g., comprehensive post-delivery follow-up of high risk mothers and their infants; regimen adherence and quality of life for transplant patients; long-term follow-up and rehabilitation for cardiac surgery patients; or meeting the special needs of post-menopausal women. Programs are often planned for installation and maintenance over extended periods, often many years. Projects, on the other hand, may be initiated to simply improve a malfunctioning system or install an innovation, such as developing a clinical guideline or a new documentation or patient intake procedure. The result of a project may have lasting effects, but the management of the project is of limited duration.

Programs require long-term management. APNs may find that creating and managing a program or project an ideal way to influence change and transform care. APNs are well positioned to design new programs, but may need considerable assistance or new skills to prepare the strategic and business plans for the program and to secure the necessary administrative and political support for program proposals. APNs can effect innovation through roles as program managers. Program management is more complex than operational management, particularly for a clinician, because specialists involved in the program generally do not have formal reporting relationships with the program manager. So program managers must exercise exceptional skills in leading, facilitating, coordinating, and holding individuals accountable for the successful function of the program. However, APNs, who have expert clinical skills, often possess sufficient expert power to successfully gain and retain the commitment of individuals involved in a program for change. If they also acquire effective leadership skills, they can use program management as a powerful tool for change. The principles of program management are similar to those required in service line management and other interdisciplinary teams, task forces, and committees. The skills required will be discussed in the final section of this chapter.

Fagin and Schwartz (1993) indicated that collaboration between nurses and physicians is "no longer a choice" (p. 8). Demonstration projects and research have demonstrated that APNs and physicians can deliver care collaboratively in an equally or more cost-effective and satisfactory fashion as either can alone. In a managed care environment, APN-physician collaboration is an important option for delivering quality health services. However, tension continues to prevent a whole-hearted acceptance of collaborative APN-physician practice. The burden of building collaborative practice with physicians has traditionally fallen to APNs, and in many cases efforts have not resulted in mutual collegiality and reciprocity. The issue of control over practice for both the APN and physician continues to prevent full implementation of collaborative practice.

The goal of APN-physician partnership is an important dimension of health care reform. Together, APNs and primary and specialist physicians can improve access and provide preventive health services as well as cost-effective management of many common and chronic illnesses. APNs will expand their roles in the future by entering into new types of community, business, and practice partnerships with physicians. As part of care delivery networks, APNs will work in mutual referral relationships with physicians and other health professionals to create new provider alliances.

With the increasing complexity of health care organizations, APNs may find significant opportunities for change agency in analyzing and improving care systems. The tools of total quality improvement may be employed by APNs and their colleagues to investigate the causes and consequences of dysfunctional organizational, administrative, and operational procedures that interfere with quality clinical service to patients and families. As APNs build stronger partnerships with administrators, managers, and physicians, they will influence the priorities given to revamping systems of admission, registration, medication management, communication, information processing, and scheduling and conduct of diagnostic procedures. APNs often have direct knowledge of patient experiences that resulted in frustration, miscommunication, lack of coordination, communication, and conflict. APNs who use quality improvement strategies can be instrumental in defining systems problems and rallying the appropriate stakeholders (managerial and clinical) to correct costly inefficiencies.

CHANGE AGENT SKILLS

Barker (1990) advocates resilience, flexibility, creativity, and responsiveness in shaping change. If change is ongoing, inevitable, and inherently patterned in health care, then the relationship of individuals involved in changing services and systems must also reflect resilience, flexibility, creativity, and highly astute observation. To effect change in a transforming health care environment, APNs must perfect skills in organizational politics, interpersonal influence, group leadership and decision making, collaboration and conflict management, systems thinking, quality improvement, and program planning and management. The acquisition of organizational skills may seem to place inordinate demands on the preparation and ongoing professional development of APNs. However, reorganized health care organizations will employ fewer managers in traditional administrative positions, and individuals with clinical and technical expertise will be thrust into leadership positions to carry out a variety of organizational initiatives.

Advanced practice nursing curriculum should include content and experiences that build knowledge and skills in exercising one-to-one, group, organizational, and community power and influence; using continuous quality improvement methods, including systems analysis; planning, organizing, and managing projects and programs; basic budgeting and business management; fundamentals of personnel supervision; group leadership and decision making; and systems analysis. APNs should be educated in strategies for developing and using organizational and community resources to build their change agent skills on an ongoing basis. Vezeau, Peterson, Nakao, and Ersek (1998) described an innovative MS in nursing curriculum aimed at preparing a Community Health Clinical Nurse Specialist Among Vulnerable Populations. One of the key concepts driving the curriculum of this program is community partnership. APNs graduating from this program will have the skills to work with members of underserved communities to identify health needs and work with them to plan programming to improve their health.

SUMMARY

The roles of APNs as future change agents is rich with possibilities, both for providing essential, quality health care services to broader sectors of the population, and for influencing the quality and cost-effectiveness of care delivery. As APNs move into new roles and as yet undefined care settings, they should possess a strong package of leadership as well as clinical skills. The skills that APNs must master if they are to be fully effective change agents include the ability to influence and build collaborative relationships with administrators, other health care providers, insurers, and community leaders, as well as to promote their innovative ideas to improve the quality and efficiency of health services for individuals and their families.

REFERENCES

Aiken, L. H., Lake, E. T., Semaan, S., Lehman, H. P., O'Hare, P. A., Cole, C. S., Dunbar, D., & Frank, L. (1993). Nurse practitioner managed care for persons with HIV infection. *Image, 25,* 172–177.

Barker, A. M. (1990). *Transformational nursing leadership: A vision for the future.* Baltimore: Williams and Wilkins.

Bissinger, R. L., Allred, C. A., Arford, D. H, & Bellig, L. L. (1997). A cost effective analysis of neonatal practitioners. *Nursing Economics, 15*(2), 92–9.

Daft, R. L. (1986). *Organization theory and design* (2nd ed.). St Paul, MN: West.

Ervin, N. E., & Young, W. B. (1996). Model for a nursing center: Spanning boundaries to improve care and service. *Journal of Nursing Care Quality, 11,* 16–24.

Fagin, C., & Schwarz, M. R. (1993). Can APNs be independent gatekeepers? *Hospitals & Health Networks, 67,* p. 8.

Finkler, M. D., & Wirtschafter, D. D. (1993). Cost-effectiveness and data envelopment analysis. *Health Care Management Review, 18,* 81–8.

Freudenheim, M. (1997, November 2). The future wears white: Nurses treading on doctors' turf. *The New York Times,* 4, 5:3.

Gibson, J. L., Ivancevich, J. M., & Donnelly, J. H., Jr. (1982). *Organizations: Behavior, structure, processes* (4th ed.). Plano, TX: Business Publications.

Hamric, A. B., & Spross, J. A. (1989). *The clinical nurse specialist in theory and practice* (2nd ed.). Philadelphia: Saunders.

Hamric, A. B., & Taylor, J. W. (1989). Role development of the CNS. In A. B. Hamric and J. A. Spross (Eds.) *The clinical nurse specialist in theory and practice* (2nd ed., pp. 41–82). Philadelphia: Saunders.

Havelock, R. (1973). *The change agent's guide to innovation in education.* New Jersey: Educational Technology Publications.

Hermann, M. K., Alexander, J. S., & Kiely, J. T. (1992). Leadership and project management. In P. J. Decker & E. J. Sullivan (Eds.), *Nursing administration: A micro-macro approach for effective nurse executives (pp.* 569–590). Norwalk, CT: Appleton & Lange.

Kaluzny, A. D., & Hernandez, S. R. (1988). Organizational change and innovation. In S. M. Shortell & A. D. Kaluzny (Eds.), *Health care management: A text in organizational theory and behavior* (2nd ed., pp. 374–417). Albany, NY: Delmar.

Kanter, R. M. (1983). *The change masters: Innovation & entrepreneurship in the American corporation.* New York: Simon and Schuster.

Keane, A., & Richmond, T. (1993). Tertiary nurse practitioners. *Image, 25,* 281–284.

Krcmar, C. R. (1991). Organizational entry: The case of the clinical nurse specialist. *Clinical Nurse Specialist, 5,* 38–42.

Lewin, K. (1958). Group decision and social change. In E. Maccoby (Ed.), *Readings in social psychology* (3rd ed.). New York: Holt, Rinehart and Winston.

Lippitt, G. (1973). *Visualizing change: Model building and the change process.* LaJolla, CA: University Associates.

McDougall, G. J. (1987). The role of the clinical nurse specialist consultant in organizational development. *Clinical Nurse Specialist, 1,* 133–139.

Miller, N. (1998). Nurse-provided primary care. *Nursing Economic$, 16,* 35.

Naylor, M. D., & Brooten, D. (1993). The roles and functions of clinical nurse specialists. *Image, 25,* 73–78.

Noone, J. (1987). Planned change: Putting theory into practice. *Clinical Nurse Specialist, 1,* 25–29.

Office of Technology Assessment. (1986). *Nurse practitioners, physician assistants and certified nurse-midwives: A policy analysis.* Washington, DC: Author.

Peters, T. J., & Waterman, R. H. (1982). *In search of excellence: Lessons from America's best-run companies.* New York: Harper & Row.

Ponte, P. R., Higgins, J. M., James, J. R., Fay, M., & Madden, M. J. (1993). Development needs of advance practice nurses in a managed care environment. *Journal of Nursing Administration, 23,* 13–19.

Safriet, B. J. (1992). Health care dollars and regulatory sense: The role of advanced practice nursing. *Yale Journal of Regulation, 9,* 417–487.

Shortell, S. M., & Kaluzny, A. D. (1988). *Health care management: A text in organization theory and behavior.* New York: Delmar.

Vezau, T. M., Peterson, J. W., Nakao, C., & Ersek, M. (1998). Education of advanced practice nurses: Serving vulnerable populations. *Nursing and Health Care Perspectives, 19,* 124–131.

Walsh, K. C. (1989). Using planned change to implement a pressure sore program. *Journal of Neuroscience Nursing, 21,* 245–249.

Welch, L. B. (1990). Planned change in nursing: The theory. In E. C. Hein & M. J. Nicholson (Eds.), *Contemporary leadership behaviors: Selected readings* (3rd ed.) (pp. 209–310). Glenview, IL: Scott, Foresman.

Wheatley, M. J. (1992). *Leadership and the new science: Learning about organization. from an orderly universe.* San Francisco: Barrett-Kohler.

Young, M. E. (1988). Entering the system as a clinical specialist using the medium of the patient care conference. *Clinical Nurse Specialist, 2,* 139–142.

Chapter 12

EVALUATING THE EFFECTIVENESS OF THE ADVANCED PRACTICE NURSE

Michaelene P. Mirr, RN, PhD, CS

Evaluating the effectiveness of advanced nursing practice presents a challenge for nursing. The importance of outcome research is noted frequently in the literature, yet minimal studies have been published in the last several years. It is often difficult to measure the direct impact that advanced practice has on health outcomes, because the role leads itself toward indirect, rather than direct, patient outcomes. In this chapter, the literature and research related to the effectiveness of advanced nursing practice will be explored.

It may be helpful to acknowledge some differences in evaluation issues for nurses in advanced practice. Historically, evaluation issues for clinical nurse specialists and nurse practitioners have been somewhat different. Clinical nurse specialists (CNSs) in hospital settings have often had to justify their positions during times of budget constraints. The CNS works or consults with a variety of individuals to attain quality standards of care. Clinical nurse specialists have struggled to find methods to measure client outcomes, as CNS's often work indirectly with clients. Since the late 1980s, more research has been conducted to quantify the impact of CNSs on the quality of care for patients and families.

Nurse practitioners, on the other hand, commonly work in joint or collaborative practice settings with physicians. Early studies attempted to justify nurse practitioner employment by comparing the care of clients under each type of care provider. Recent studies have examined the effectiveness of prescribing practices by APNs (Cornwell & Chiverton, 1997; Hamric, Worley, Lindebak, & Jaubert, 1998)

Several comprehensive reviews of research studies examining the effectiveness of clinical nurse specialists and nurse practitioners have been conducted (Crosby, Ventura, & Feldman, 1987; Feldman, Ventura, & Crosby, 1987; Naylor & Brooten, 1993; Office of Technology Assessment, 1986; Werner, Bumann, & O'Brien, 1989). These reviews make a clear distinction between performance appraisal and impact on quality care. This chapter focuses on how the APN can improve patient and family care outcomes in a fiscally responsible way. Therefore, three categories of evaluation research will be discussed: time documentation, comparison of advanced practice nurse effectiveness, and care outcomes.

As research on the effectiveness of advanced practice has evolved, so has the health care system. Effectiveness of advanced nursing practice often translates into cost-effectiveness. Cost-effectiveness is currently the outcome assuming major importance. Ahrens and Padwojski (1988) noted that it is difficult to convert impact on quality care into economic impact terms.

EVALUATION VARIABLE

Time Involvement

Time documentation is one type of structural evaluation measure that can be used to determine whether or not an advanced practice nurse is able to effectively prioritize and categorize time to make an impact on patient and family care (Robichaud & Hamric, 1986). Hamric (1989) stated that nurses in advanced practice have a tendency to move too quickly to outcome measures before they are able to effectively prioritize and organize time. Time documentation is helpful for nurses new to advanced practice to develop their roles efficiently and effectively. Experienced APNs can also use time documentation to redirect focus of practice due to changing environmental and patient needs (Robichaud & Hamric, 1986).

Robichaud and Hamric (1986) caution that time documentation alone is insufficient as a means of measuring the impact of practice. The main limitation of time documentation studies is that they do not provide a direct measurement of the APN's effectiveness (Hamric, 1989). For example, an APN may take 15 extra minutes to reinforce teaching a diabetic how to identify early signs of insulin reaction. A time study would show that in the short term, the APN was inefficient; but in terms of long-term outcomes, the extra time may prevent an emergency room admission. Safriet (1992) encouraged examining time in relation to long-term outcomes.

One of the earliest documented time studies determined that during the first year of practice, CNSs concentrated their time on direct patient care, whereas experienced CNSs devoted their time to education, community activities, and consultation (Aradine & Denyes, 1972). Other time documentation studies validated that clinical nurse specialists spend between 40–50% of their time on direct patient care (Burge, Crigler, Hurth, Kelly, & Sanborn, 1989; Robichaud & Hamric, 1986; Wright, Owen, Murphy, Kenning, & Grenshaw, 1984). The main implication of time documentation studies is that as the CNS develops his or her role, a decreased portion of that role is devoted to direct patient care. Rather, the CNS functions within a broader, more community-based focus.

Productivity tools for nurse practitioners have historically been limited to evaluation of the number of patient visits or amount of revenue generated. The proliferation of MCOs has emphasized productivity. Keames (1992) argued that such instruments do not always reflect the amount of time spent with the patient or delineate between patient time, travel time, and administrative time. Keames proposed a computerized system that assigns a weight to each patient visit based on duration of visit, in order to determine productive time rather than administrative or travel time. This system provides a classification system to determine whether the nurse practitioner is attaining an ideal productivity level. However, the evaluation will differ, depending on whether it is viewed from a long-term or short-term outcome perspective.

Advanced Practice Nurse-Physician Effectiveness

Whereas early studies of clinical nurse specialists have focused on time documentation studies, early research on the effectiveness of nurse practitioners centered on comparisons of nurse practitioner and physician care. Many studies regarding the effectiveness of nurse practitioners and certified nurse midwives have compared their productivity, ability, and patient satisfaction with those of physicians. The Office of Technology and Assessment (OTA) (1986) concluded that nurse practitioners possessed the knowledge and expertise to meet the health needs of 50–90% of the ambulatory care patient population. The report cited 10 studies that demonstrated that patient care provided by nurse practitioners and physicians was equivalent. Although the OTA recognized some methodological problems with these studies, it concluded that nurse practitioners were more cost-effective and accessible than their physician counterparts in providing care to the majority of ambulatory care clients. Nurse practitioners spent more time with patients, saw fewer patients, and cost approximately 20% less than physicians (Nichols, 1992; Safriet, 1992). The decreased caseload can be justified because nurse practitioners provide a broader spectrum of services.

Many studies comparing physicians and nurse practitioners have been retrospective chart reviews (Campbell, Mauksch, Neikirk, & Hosokawa, 1990; Diers, Hamman, & Molde, 1986; Hall et al., 1990; Melillo, 1990). Campbell et al. (1990) found few differences in the interaction styles of nurse practitioners and physicians. These authors demonstrated that patient-provider interactions could be measured and that these interactions may influence the direction of patient outcomes.

The caseloads of master's-prepared nurse practitioners, attending physicians, and resident physicians at an inner city teaching hospital were compared in a study conducted by Diers et al. (1986). The study found that NPs saw more non-White and public assistance patients than the attending and resident physicians. Patients seen by nurse practitioners frequently had multiple problems, minor injuries or illnesses, and slightly higher admission rates. Physician-generated patient records often lacked social data, such as information about the patient's living conditions and occupation. Although there were no differences in use of health care services by each group, the physicians tended to prescribe more medications.

Another study examined differences in quality of medical care based on gender of health care providers and gender of patients (Hall et al., 1990). Comparisons were made between physicians and nonphysicians (nurse practitioners and physician assistants). The investigators conducted a chart review of eight common conditions. Findings suggested that female NPs, with the exception of cancer screening, gave care comparable and sometimes superior to that provided by staff and resident physicians. Data from this study indicated that patients of the gender most commonly associated with a condition received better care. There were no differences in quality of care provided by NPs who consulted physicians frequently as compared to those who consulted physicians infrequently.

As more states allow independent prescribing practices for APNs, comparison studies between prescribing practices of physicians and advanced practice nurses are beginning to emerge. Hamric, Worley, Lindebak & Jaubert (1998) examined outcomes related to prescribing practices between physicians and APNs. They evaluated the safety and effectiveness of the APNs prescriptive authority using three different outcome measures: patient outcome, patient assessment of outcome, and physician assessment of outcome. The authors found that APNs were safe and effective in their prescribing practices.

Comparisons of NPs and physicians have also been conducted in long-term care facilities. A retrospective chart audit on 2651 long-term care patients in 110 nursing homes was conducted by Melillo (1990). Comparisons were made with the process and outcomes of traditional medical care. The findings indicated that patients cared for by nurse practitioners had less functional impairments.

Other studies comparing NPs and physicians used interviews to determine differences and similarities of care (McClain, 1985; Powers, Jalowiec, & Reichelt, 1984; Salisbury & Tettersell, 1988). McClain's phenomenological study explored factors which prevent meaningful collaboration between physicians, nurse practitioners, and clients. Only a few of the 18 NP–MD teams studied were found to be truly collaborative. Characteristics common to collaborative teams included sincerity and comprehensiveness, as well as the ability to clarify situations or misperceptions.

To determine patient knowledge, satisfaction, compliance, and problem resolution in nonurgent emergency department patients, Powers et al., (1984) randomly assigned 62 patients to a nurse practitioner or a physician. Outcomes were measured following the visit, at 2-week and 3-month intervals. No significant differences between physicians and NPs were found related to outcomes of knowledge, satisfaction and compliance, and problem resolution. Patients seen by NPs reported more overall satisfaction with care received.

Salisbury & Tettersell (1988) compared workloads of nurse practitioners and general practice physicians in Great Britain. Nurse practitioners primarily managed patients with chronic conditions such as diabetes, hypertension, and obesity. Nurse practitioners wrote prescriptions for 11% of the patients compared to 57% for physicians. Patients cited several reasons for choosing nurse practitioners, including the ease of talking with nurses and the greater accessibility of nurses. The authors concluded that NPs placed more emphasis on practical health care services than did physicians.

Care Outcomes

The growing emphasis on quality and cost-effective care has shifted the research emphasis from time documentation and determination of APN effectiveness toward care outcomes and cost-effectiveness. Research examining patient and family outcomes provides qualitative and quantitative data regarding quality care as well as cost-effectiveness.

Some of the earliest data were obtained by Brooten et al. (1986). Brooten and colleagues examined the effects of early hospital discharge and home follow-up by an advanced practice nurse on very low birth weight infants. Families in the early discharge group received instruction, counseling, and home visits, as well as on-call availability of the perinatal nurse specialist. Hospital and physician charges for the experimental group were 27% and 22% less, respectively, when compared to the control group. No significant differences in the number of rehospitalizations, acute care visits, or developmental outcomes between the two groups were found.

Based on their research, Brooten and colleagues have developed a model, "Quality Cost Model of Clinical Specialist Transitional Care," as a framework that can be applied to any hospitalized patient population at risk for poor postdischarge outcomes (Brooten et al., 1988). The model has been tested on women with unplanned Cesarean births, pregnant diabetic women, post-hysterectomy patients, children with AIDS, and elderly (Naylor & Brooten, 1993). The model is unique in that it addresses APNs and is neither CNS- nor NP-specific.

The Brooten model utilizes a comprehensive program of transitional home follow-up provided by advanced practice nurses. The model is illustrated in Table 12.1 and offers APNs a model to use in their own practices. Brooten et al. (1988) define transitional follow-up care as "care from discharge planning through the period of normally expected physiologic recovery" (p. 66). Patients and families are included in this program if they meet specific criteria for early discharge. Early discharge accounts for approximately a 20% decrease in length of hospital stay. The APN prepares the patient for discharge, coordinates teaching, schedules the time of discharge, establishes community referrals, and schedules medical follow-up. Following discharge, the APN makes a

TABLE 12.1   Quality-Cost of Early Hospital Discharge and Nurse Specialist Transitional Follow-up Care

Hospitalization	Post-Discharge	End of Normal Convalescent Period
Early Discharge	*Intervention*	*Quality*
Women with Common Life Events or Situational Crisis	Transitional follow-up by nurse specialists via preparation for discharge, home visits, telephone contact and daily availability	Patient Outcomes Physical -Morbidity–infection, acute care visits, rehospitalization Psychosocial
Preparation for 3 Groups Discharge		-Anxiety -Depression
1. Unplanned Patient Cesarean a. Physical Birth b. Emotional 2. Childbearing c. Knowledge base 3. Women Environmental having adequacy hysterectomies Coordination of discharge planning	Home Visits Telephone Contacts & Daily Nurse Available by Telephone	-Hostility -Self-esteem -Satisfaction with care
		Cost Cost of Care -Initial hospitalization -Physician services
	Assessment and monitoring of patient physical and emotional status, provisions of direct care as needed, assessment of environmental support & assistance in obtaining community resources where needed, teaching and counseling	-Nurse specialist services -Time lost from employment by family members assuming care during early discharge period
		Quality Patient Outcomes Physical -Mobility-infection, acute care visits, rehospitalization -Return to normal activities Psychosocial -Anxiety -Depression -Hostility -Self-esteem -Satisfaction with care
Routine Discharge Women with Common Life Events or Situational Crisis 3 Groups 1. Unplanned Cesarean birth 2. Childbearing diabetics 3. Women having hysterectomies		Cost Cost of Care -Initial hospitalization -Rehospitalization -Physician services -Nurse specialist services -Time lost from employment by family members assuming care during early discharge period

Brown, B. M. Margo, R. York, S. M. Cohen, H. Roncoli, & A. Hallingsworth. (1988). Image: Journal of Nursing Scholarship, 20 pp. 64–68. Copyright 1988 by Sigma Theta Tau International. With permission of Sigma Theta Tau International.

series of home visits and communicates frequently with the patient and family via telephone to "assess and monitor the physical, emotional and functional status of the patient, provide direct care when needed, assist in obtaining services or other resources available in the community, and provide group specific teaching, counseling and support during the period of convalescence" (p. 67).

Brooten and colleagues (1988) distinguish this program from other discharge planning programs in that clinical specialists are master's-prepared and possess specific knowledge and expertise in a particular area of patient care. Another strength of this model is that it allows teaching and counseling to be provided by the same professional over an extended period of time. Brooten and colleagues suggest that if institutions do not have a large enough caseload to support this model, community health agencies may subcontract to provide follow-up care for specific client groups.

Another study in transitional care was conducted by Neidlinger, Scroggins, and Kennedy (1987) to determine the cost-effectiveness of a comprehensive hospital discharge planning program for patients over 75 years old that was coordinated by a gerontological clinical nurse specialist. Subjects were randomly assigned to an experimental or control group for 4 weeks. Findings indicate that the average daily hospital cost for the experimental group was $60.00 less than the control group, yielding a net savings of $34,707 during the 4-week study period.

Other studies have demonstrated that education and early involvement with children with chronic illness by APNs have decreased the length of hospital stays and decreased hospital or emergency visits (Alexander, Younger, Cohen, & Crawford, 1988; Lipman, 1986). The post-myocardial infarction population has also benefited from APN intervention. Two studies have demonstrated that when a CNS provided education and was involved in care, patients returned earlier to work and had decreased psychological stress (Burgess, Lemer, D'Agostino, Vokonas, Hartman, & Gaccione, 1987; Pozen et al., 1977). Urban (1997) documented a decrease in the length of stay of 2–9 days and a 58% reduction in complications utilizing an APN in a cardiovascular acute care setting. A multidisciplinary collaboration practice model utilizing a critical care APN in a surgical intensive care unit (SICU) produced a $157,000 cost savings and a decrease in length of stay of 1.4 days.

Formulas to determine the cost-effectiveness of employing nurse practitioners within a medical practice have been developed. It is estimated that a nurse practitioner can handle 63% of a physician's caseload at 38% of the cost, resulting in an overall savings of 24% (McGrath, 1990; Poirier-Elliott, 1984; Record, McCally, Schweitzer, Blomquist, & Berger, 1980; Sweet, 1986). Nichols (1992) designed a model for estimating the actual costs of underutilization rather than using a model based on potential savings. Nichols notes that actual estimates may be more persuasive to policymakers. The cost-effectiveness of the nurse practitioner, however, has not been fully actualized due to numerous legislative, social, and reimbursement restrictions (McGrath, 1990; Sullivan, 1992; Sweet, 1986).

Cost-effectiveness cannot always be associated with consumer satisfaction or quality care. Careful critique of research is essential to determine the quality of the study conducted. For example, Feldman et al. (1987) conducted an analysis of research literature on nurse practitioners. Of the 248 documents reviewed, 56 met the validity and reliability criteria determined by the authors. The conclusions of this analysis demonstrate consumer satisfaction with nurse practitioners without loss of quality of care.

Touger & Butts (1989) examined outcomes of a health care center staffed by APNs. Nurse practitioners and support staff provided primary health care for the employees, which included diagnosis and treatment of acute problems, counseling, referrals, and wellness programs. A family practice physician provided consultative services to the center. In addition to large insurance cost savings, the program was beneficial because employees spent less time away from work and acquired increased self-care skills.

An important aspect of nursing is health promotion and health prevention. However, our health care system and billing mechanisms have put little emphasis on this, and few studies have been conducted. Snow, Calder, Taylor, Lane, and Federici (1989) reported outcomes from a preventive health program that screened for lung, colon, skin, and prostate/breast cancer. Over a 1-year period, 176 patients at a Veterans Administration Center were referred and randomly evaluated. During this time, six cancers were confirmed, and 57% of the patients were diagnosed with hypercholesterolemia. Of these, 19% were found to have three or more risk factors for coronary artery disease. The authors concluded that cost savings from early intervention far outweighed the cost of screening.

Teaching nursing homes, where faculty prepared as clinical nurse specialists and nurse practitioners and students provided direct care to nursing home residents, have demonstrated positive client outcomes (Aiken, Mezey, Lynaugh, & Buck, 1985; Mezey & Lynaugh, 1989). Residents of these facilities had decreased hospital admissions and increased quality of care. Quality of care was measured in terms of increased functional abilities, decreased incidence of incontinence, appropriate use of medications, and decreased use of chemical and physical restraints.

Advanced Nursing Functions

A recent trend in advanced practice research has been to examine APN functions in an attempt to define and demonstrate the unique APN role (Naylor & Brooten, 1993). The APN's job description plays a vital role in evaluating outcomes based on APN functions. Job descriptions are often used to determine and measure expected outcomes. Incongruencies in job descriptions can decrease the ability for APNs to document their activities, thus leading to expectations or outcomes that are not met.

IMPLICATIONS FOR FURTHER RESEARCH

To determine what is needed in the future in terms of APN research, one can ask the question, "What do we know and what is critical in the next decade?" Research has demonstrated that APNs can provide safe and effective care for the majority of ambulatory care patients in a cost-effective manner. Several studies have demonstrated significant cost savings related to interventions by APNs. However, these studies are only a beginning in what is needed to document the contributions of APNs. The lack of recent studies addressing APN effectiveness based on long-term outcomes, as well as an examination of the cost-effectiveness of APNs based on the mix of nurse and physician providers in a variety of settings, suggests that APNs need to move beyond previous laurels and begin documenting this effectiveness (Sherwood, Brown, Fay, & Wardell, 1997).

Research on the effectiveness of APNs is challenging because many APN functions are collaborative and difficult to measure directly. Munro (1993) refers to a National Institute of Nursing Research Conference on patient outcome research which recommended implementation of an organized approach to patient outcome research. Research on the effectiveness of all APN types (NP, CNS, CRNA, CNM) is needed (Crosby et al., 1987; Naylor & Brooten, 1993; Sherwood et al., 1997). Research related to the effectiveness of APNs will need to be designed well, use outcome variables that reflect the care provided, and demonstrate cost-effectiveness.

REFERENCES

Ahrens, T., & Padwojski, A. (1988). Economic impact of advanced clinicians. *Nursing Management 19*, 64A-64F.

Aiken, L., Mezey, M., Lynaugh, J. E., & Buck, C. R. (1985). Teaching nursing homes: Prospects for improving long term care. *Journal of the American Gerontological Association, 33*, 196–201.

Alexander, J. S., Younger, R. E., Cohen, R. M., & Crawford, J. (1988). Effectiveness of a nurse managed program for children with chronic asthma. *Journal of Pediatric Nursing, 3*, 312–317.

Aradine, C. R., & Denyes, M. J. (1972). Activities and pressures of clinical nurse specialists. *Nursing Research, 21*, 411–418.

Brooten, D., Brown, L. P., Munro, B. H., York, R., Cohen, S. M., Roncoli,M., & Hollingsworth, A. (1988). Early discharge and specialist transitional care. *Image: Journal of Nursing Scholarship, 20*, 64–68.

Brooten, D., Kumar, S., Butts, P., Finkler, S., Bakewell-Sach, S., Gibbons, A., & Delivoria-Papadopoulos, M. (1986). A randomized clinical trial of early hospital discharge and home follow-up of very low birthweight infants. *New England Journal of Medicine, 315*, 934–939.

Buhler, L., Glick, N., & Sheps, S. B. (1988). Prenatal care: A comparative evaluation of nurse-midwives and family physicians. *Canadian Media Association Journal, 139*, 397–403.

Burge, S., Crigler, L., Hurth, L., Kelly, G., & Sanborn, C. (1989). Clinical Nurse Specialist Role Development: Quantifying actual practice over three years. *Clinical Nurse Specialist, 3*, 33–36.

Burgess, A. W., Lemer, D. J., D'Agostino, R. B., Vokonas, P. S., C.R., & Gaccione, P. (1987). A randomized control trial of cardiac rehabilitation. *Social Science Medicine, 24*, 359–370.

Campbell, J. D., Mauksch, H. O., Neikirk, H. J., & Hosokawa, M. (1990) Collaborative practice and provider styles of delivering health care. *Social Science and Medicine, 30*, 1359–1365.

Cornwell, C. & Chiverton, P. (1997). The psychiatric advanced practice nurse with prescriptive authority: Role development, practice issues, and outcome measurements. *Archives of Psychiatric Nursing, 11*(2), 57–65.

Crosby, F., Ventura, M. R., & Feldman, M. J. (1987). Future research recommendations for establishing NP effectiveness. *Nurse Practitioner, 12,* 75–79.

Diers, D., Hamman, A., & Molde, S. (1986). Complexity of ambulatory care: Nurse practitioner and physician caseloads. *Nursing Research, 35,* 310–314.

Donabedian, A. (1966). Evaluating the quality of medical care. *Milbank Memorial Fund Quarterly, 44,* 166–206.

Feldman, M. J., Ventura, M., & Crosby, F. (1987). Studies of nurse practitioner effectiveness. *Nursing Research, 36,* 303–308.

Hall, J. A., Palmer, R. H., Orav, E. J., Hargraves, J. L., Wright, E. A. 9 & Louis, T. A. (1990). Performance quality, gender and professional role: A study of physician and nonphysicians in 16 ambulatory care practices. *Medical Care, 28,* 489–501.

Hamric, A. B. (1989). A model for CNS evaluation. In A. B. Hamric & J. Spross (Eds.), *77ze clinical nurse specialist in theory and practice* (2nd ed.). (pp. 83–104). Philadelphia: W.B. Saunders.

Hamric, A.B., Worley, D., Lindebak, S., & Jaubert, S. (1997). Outcomes associated with advanced practice prescriptive authority. *Journal of the American Academy of Nurse Practitioners, 10*(3), 113–118.

Keames, D. R. (1992). A productivity tool to evaluate NP practice: Monitoring clinical time spent in reimbursable patient-related activities. *Nurse Practitioner, 17, 50–55.*

Lamb, G. S. (1991). Two explanations of nurse practitioner interactions and participatory decision making with physicians. *Research in Nursing & Health, 14,* 379–386.

Lipman, T. (1986). Length of hospitalization of children with diabetes: Effect of a clinical nurse specialist. The *Diabetes Educator, 14,* 41–43.

Mahoney, D. F. (1988). An economic analysis of the nurse practitioner role. *Nurse Practitioner, 13,* 44–45, 48–52.

McAlpine, L.A. (1997). Process and outcome measures for the multidisciplinary collaborative projects of a critical care CNS. *Clinical Nurse Specialist, 11*(3), 134–138.

McClain, B. R. (1985). Patterns of interaction, decision-making and health care delivery by nurse practitioners and physicians in joint practice. *Dissertation Abstracts International, 47,* 3295B. (University Microfilms No. ACC8628340).

McCormick, K. A. (1991). Future data needs for quality of care monitoring, DRG considerations, reimbursement and outcome measurement. Image: *Journal of Nursing Scholarship, 23,* 29–32.

McGrath, S. (1990). The cost-effectiveness of nurse practitioners. *Nurse Practitioner, 15,* 40–42.

Melillo, K. D. (1990). Evaluation of nursing process and outcomes of care utilizing nurse practitioners to provide health care for elderly patients in

Massachusetts nursing homes. *Dissertations Abstracts International, 51,* 3780B. (University Microfilms No. DA9100460).

Mezey, M., & Lynaugh, J. (1989). The teaching nursing home program: Outcomes of care. *Nursing Clinics of North America, 24,* 769–780.

Molde, S., & Diers, D. (1985). Nurse practitioner research: Selected literature review and research agenda. *Nursing Research, 34,* 362–367.

Munro, B. H. (1993). Measuring outcomes of our practice. *Clinical Nurse Specialist, 7*(5), 246.

Naylor, M. D., & Brooten, D. (1993). The roles and functions of clinical nurse specialists. *Image: Journal of Nursing Scholarship, 25,* 73–78.

Neidlinger, S. H., Scroggins, K., & Kennedy, L. M. (1987). Cost evaluation of discharge planning for hospitalized elderly. *Nursing Economics, 5,* 225–230.

Nichols, L. M. (1992). Estimating costs of underusing advanced practice nurses. *Nursing Economics, 10,* 343–351.

Office of Technology Assessment. (1986). *Nurse practitioners, physician assistants, and certified nurse midwives: A policy analysis.* (Health Technology Care Study 37, OTA-HCS-37). Washington, DC: U.S. Government Printing Office.

Peglow, D. M., Klatt-Ellis, T., Stelton, S., Cutillo-Schmitter, T., Howard, J., & Wolff, P. (1992). Evaluation of clinical nurse specialist pracatice. *Clinical Nurse Specialist, 6,* 28–35.

Poirier-Elliot, E. (1984). Cost-effectiveness of non-physician healthcare professionals. *Nurse Practitioner, 9,* 54–56.

Powers, M. J., Jalowiec, A., & Reichelt, P. A. (1984). Nurse practitioner and physician care compared for non urgent emergency room patients. *Nurse Practitioner, 9,* 39–52.

Pozen, M. N., Stechmiller, J. A., Harris, W. A., Smith, S., Fried, D. D., & Voight, G. C. (1977). A nurse rehabilitator's impact on patients with myocardial infarction. *Medical Care, 15,* 830–837.

Record, J. C., McCally, M., Schweitzer, S. O., Blomquist, R. M., & Berger, B. D. (1980). New health professionals after a decade and a half. *Journal of Health, Politics, Policy, and Law, 5,* 470–497.

Robichaud, A. M., & Hamric, A. (1986). Time documentation of clinical nurse specialist activities. *Journal of Nursing Administration, 16,* 31–36.

Safriet, B. J. (1992). Health care dollars and regulatory sense: The role of Advanced Practice Nursing. *Yale Journal on Regulation, 9,* 419–487.

Salisbury, C. J., & Tettersell, M. J. (1988). Comparison of the work of a nurse practitioner with that of a general practitioner. *Journal of the Royal College of General Practitioners, 38,* 314–316.

Sherwood, G. S., Brown, M., Fay, V., & Wardell, D. (1997). Defining nurse practitioner scope of practice: Expanding primary care services. *Internet Journal of Advanced Nursing Practice 1*(2) [On-line.] Available: http://www.ispub.com/journals/IJAPN/vol1N2/scope.htm.

Snow, S. G., Calder, E. A., Taylor, L. S., Lane, T. J., & Federici, C. M. (1989).

Screening for cancer and coronary risk factors through a nurse practitioner-staffed preventive health clinic. *Preventive Medicine, 13,* 236–241.

Sullivan, E. M. (1992). Nurse practitioners and reimbursement. *Nursing and Health Care, 13,* 236–41.

Sweet, J. B. (1986). The cost-effectiveness of nurse practitioners. *Nursing Economics, 4.* 190–193.

Touger, G. N., & Butts, J. K. (1989). The workplace: An innovative and cost effective practice site. *Nurse Practitioner, 14,* 35–42.

Urban, N. (1997). Managed care challenges and opportunities for cardiovascular advanced practice nurses. *AACN Clinical Issues, 8,* 78–89.

Werner, J. S., Bumann, R. M., & O'Brien, J. A. (1989). Clinical nurse specialization: An annotated bibliography: Evaluation and impact. *Clinical Nurse Specialist, 3,* 20–36.

Wright, L., Owen, J., Murphy, K., Kenning, D., & Grenshaw, C. (1984). Capsule: A profile for clinical nurse specialists. *The Journal of Nursing Administration, 14,* 36.

Chapter 13

PROFESSIONAL COMMUNICATION: PUBLISHING AND PRESENTATIONS

Mariah Snyder, PhD, RN, FAAN

Communication plays an important role in nursing. Effective interpersonal communication has been recognized for many years as a characteristic of good nursing practice (Ryden, 1998). Because skillful interpersonal interactions convey the nurse's interest in and concern for the person, clients possess a high trust in nurses. Because of this trust, clients readily share a considerable amount of information about themselves that assists nurses to make diagnoses and implement effective care plans. For Advance Practice Nurses (APN), effective interpersonal skills are key in obtaining assessment data, developing a plan of care in collaboration with the patient, and in using interpersonal techniques as interventions.

Another aspect of communication to which nurses have given less attention is the sharing of information with colleagues, other professionals, and the public. This sharing is done via many avenues including articles in nursing journals, interdisciplinary journals and lay publications; written teaching materials; oral and poster presentations at nursing, interdisciplinary, and community meetings; and interviews for radio, television, or newspapers. Publications and presentations will be discussed in this chapter.

Sharing of information with peers is necessary if nursing is to develop a substantive basis for its practice and to improve nursing practice. Exchanges allow others to know what has proven to be successful and what remains to be studied. In this age of communication it is also imperative that nurses provide the public arena with knowledge about nursing's contributions to positive health outcomes. APNs assume a major role in communicating practice findings to various audiences. The recent positive media presentations about APNs, such as on *60 Minutes,* have provided magnificent opportunities for increasing the public's awareness about APNs.

PUBLISHING

A characteristic of a profession is that it has an established body of knowledge. Traditionally nurses have placed emphasis on "doing" and not on pondering and thinking. When queried, many nurses in clinical settings state that they are "too busy" to write. Others feel that they lack the skills necessary to develop a manuscript for publication. The merit system in clinical settings often does not include publications as a criterion, so nurses in clinical agencies have not been encouraged to publish. If nursing as a profession is to advance, it is incumbent on APNs to publish. According to Styles (1978), "The primary reason to publish is because the future of the profession depends upon it" (p. 29).

A phenomenal increase in the number of nursing journals has occurred during the past two decades. Swanson, McCloskey, and Bodensteiner (1991) conducted an extensive review of the literature to determine existing nursing journals. Ninety-two nursing journals were identified in 1991, as compared to only 22 that were in existence in 1977. McConnell (1995) identified 102 nursing journals published outside of the United States.

For persons who feel that they do not possess the skills or knowledge necessary to publish, numerous books and articles provide specific guidance for the neophyte. Some of these are *Publication Manual of the American Psychological Association* (American Psychological Association, 1994); *Secrets of Successful Writing* (Scott, 1989); *Watch Your Language* (Zorn, Smith, & Werley, 1991); *A Practice Guide to Writing for Publication* (Robinson, Collins, & Monkman, 1997); *The Publication Process: Steps to Success* (Tucker-Allen, 1997); *Writing of Publica-*

tion: Understanding the Process (Plawecki & Plawecki, 1998); *Writing Tips for Authors* (Servodidio, 1998); *Writing and Getting Published* (Barnum, 1995); and *How to Write and Publish Articles in Nursing, 2nd Edition* (Sheridan & Dowdney, 1997).

Initial Strategies

APNs possess a vast store of information to share with colleagues and with the public. A few of the areas in which APNs are very knowledgeable include research or evaluation studies that have been conducted, literature reviews that were done prior to developing a protocol, descriptions of a new role or practice, strategies that have been used to market a new product or practice, changes in the health care system and how these affect nursing, and issues facing the profession. It should not take an APN much time identify a topic or topics about which she/he has expertise that could be shared with colleagues.

Sometimes nurses feel reluctant to venture alone in developing a manuscript. As can be noted when reviewing nursing journals, the majority of articles have multiple authors. Working with colleagues has both advantages and disadvantages; most frequently the advantages outweigh the disadvantages. Advantages and disadvantages of working collaboratively are listed in Table 13.1. Before embarking on a collaborative publishing endeavor, participants need to establish guidelines that address the specific tasks of each member and the time frame for completing the tasks. Attention to what occurs if a person does not fulfill his or her tasks also needs to be addressed. For example, are persons dropped from the team if they fail to follow through on their commitments?

Authorship is an important aspect to clarify when collaborating with

TABLE 13.1   Advantages and Disadvantages of Joint Authorship

Advantages	Disadvantages
Encouragement	Get bogged down about
Built-in critiques	direction of manuscript
Each work on a part	Arguments about authorship
of the article	Some not doing their fair share
Have commitment to another,	
so see project to fruition	

peers in developing a manuscript. Frequently, little attention is given to this until the manuscript is finished. According to Stevens (1986), disagreements about authorship have resulted in destroying teams and ending future collaboration. "Who will be listed as an author?" and "What order will the names be listed?" are two questions that should be discussed at an early team meeting. Inclusion of a person's name as an author indicates that the individual has made substantive contributions to the project, to the writing of the manuscript, and is willing to assume public responsibility for the content of the manuscript (Midwest Nursing Research Society [MNRS], 1996). "Substantive contribution" includes two or more of the following: conception and design of the project or manuscript; execution of the project; analysis and interpretation of the data; and preparation and revision of the manuscript (MNRS). Persons who make a minor contribution to a manuscript can be acknowledged in a footnote.

The sequencing of names is more complicated than deciding who will be included in the list of authors. If one person has done the majority of the project or the writing, then that person's name should be listed first. When all persons have contributed equally to a project and the writing of the manuscript, listing the names in alphabetical order is appropriate. A footnote can indicate the basis for the listing. Most often the sequencing of authors reflects the descending order of involvement in the project (Stevens, 1986). One strategy for avoiding controversies about authorship is an agreement that a specific person will be the senior author on one manuscript, while another person will be the senior author on a subsequent manuscript.

Many projects provide opportunities for multiple manuscripts to be published. However, each publication needs to be independent, and not just duplication of content. Blancett (1991) termed this latter practice as "salami publishing." This type of publishing can include very similar manuscripts with only minor modifications, similar manuscripts prepared for journals in different disciplines, and developing multiple manuscripts when one would have sufficed (Blancett, 1991). Thus, while multiple manuscripts are often possible, authors must consider the nature of the manuscripts so as to avoid "giving everyone a chance to have her/his name as first author."

Getting Organized

One of the first decisions to be made is determining the audience who will most benefit from the information to be shared. Does the topic have wide appeal in nursing? A more general nursing journal, such as the

American Journal of Nursing, would be an appropriate vehicle for sharing information on a general topic. In contrast, the topic may be related to a specific population or setting. Thus, a clinical specialty journal or journal for a particular setting, such as *School Nurse,* should be considered. Perusing the listing of journals identified by Swanson et al. (1991) will assist nurses in selecting the most appropriate journals for submitting their manuscript.

After selecting possible journals, recent issues of the journals should be reviewed to determine if articles on the proposed topic have been recently published. Just because a similar topic has been published does not necessarily negate submission of the planned manuscript. The proposed manuscript may offer new ideas on the topic, or refute some of the information contained in a published article. However, if the proposed manuscript does not differ significantly from a recently published article, the manuscript will most likely not be considered for publication in that journal.

Submitting a query letter to the editor of a journal will provide feedback on whether the journal has similar topics under consideration for publication, and thus prevent a later rejection from that journal because the topic has been addressed. In query letters, authors describe their proposed manuscript, why it will be of interest to readers, and the author's qualifications for writing on the particular topic (Herrin, 1989). A manuscript can only be submitted to only one journal at a time, but query letters can be sent to multiple journal editors. Before sending a query letter, the authors should obtain the name of the journal editor and address the letter to the specific person. The editor's name can be found on the index page of each issue of a journal.

Determining the main focus of a manuscript is a key step. Many approaches can be used in discussing and presenting a particular topic. For example, nurses could focus on the nature of the new practice guidelines that were introduced in their setting, or the focus could be on the strategies used to initiate and implement the new practice guidelines. Identifying the audience helps the author(s) to focus on the particular approach to use in presenting the content.

Developing the introduction to the manuscript often takes time. Having an established focus assists the author in writing the introduction. Unless the lead paragraph is written in a way that "grabs" or "hooks" the reader, the subsequent content may not be read. Some authors spend considerable time on this paragraph initially, while others finalize it after they have completed the remainder of the manuscript.

Most authors develop a detailed outline for the proposed manuscript. The outline provides a vehicle for reviewing multiple ideas and determining if they are appropriate to include in this particular manuscript. The outline allows the author to establish a logical flow for the content. Developing the outline may reveal gaps in the proposed manuscript and a need to review additional literature or obtain additional background information.

Establishing a time frame for completing the manuscript is important. Having pre-established times helps to keep the project moving. Without a schedule, it is too easy to put writing off, as other activities often seem to be more urgent. Failure to adhere to the established schedule can create guilt and may serve as an impetus to "keep going."

Word processing has changed writing in many ways. Most authors feel comfortable in placing the outline next to the word processor and then begin to "write." In contrast, others feel more comfortable jotting down many thoughts in longhand before beginning to truly compose the manuscript. Some persons prefer to sit down and type/write very freely and not make corrections in the content until they have typed/written down all of the major ideas they wish to present. They then return and edit the manuscript. Others, however, prefer to get a near final product completed as they proceed. Numerous corrections are made in each paragraph as they develop the manuscript. Each author has to identify the style of writing that best fits with her/his disposition and talents.

Each journal uses a specific style or format. Directions for the specific journal are contained in many issues of the journal, or may be obtained from the journal editor or the journal's website. Because the style varies across journals, time is saved if the author is familiar with the specific guidelines when beginning to develop the manuscript. Other information that is important to obtain about publishing in a specific journal is the desired length for manuscripts; whether tables, figures, or photographs can be included; and whether a formal or lay language is used in the journal.

Manuscript

After completing a near-final product, many authors find it helpful to set aside the manuscript for a week or more and then to reread it. New ideas for ways to present content, use of language that would add clarity to ideas, and the need to rearrange content for a more logical flow of ideas may become evident after a period away from the manuscript. One aspect requiring attention when multiple persons have written sections of a manuscript is blending the various writing styles so that it appears as if it were composed by one person. This usually involves rewriting of some segments by the senior author so that the flow is consistent throughout the manuscript.

The majority of journals require an abstract to accompany the manuscript; the abstract contains the key points of the manuscript. Abstracts are very important, as they are obtained when literature searches are done. The length of the abstract varies for each journal. Composing the abstract is a good activity to do while "letting the manuscript set for a few days." Most journals request the author to identify three key words that are the chief foci of the manuscript. Careful attention to the words specified is necessary, as these are the words that will guide users to the article when literature searches are conducted.

Another practice that assists authors in submitting a manuscript that has a higher likelihood to be accepted for publication is asking colleagues to critique the manuscript. One practice is to have the manuscript critiqued by a colleague who is familiar with the content area, and have another critique done by a person who is unfamiliar with the content area. The first reviewer is able to provide feedback on vital content that may have been omitted, or indicate areas requiring further clarification. The reviewer who is unfamiliar with the content critiques the manuscript for its understandability and logical flow. This feedback assists the authors in making the final revisions of the manuscript.

Table 13.2 presents the final checklist for authors to complete before submitting a manuscript to *Geriatric Nursing*. Other journals also in-

---

TABLE 13.2   Final Check List Before Submitting the Manuscript

__ Letter of submission
__ Signed copyright transfer statement
__ Title page (three copies, double-spaced)
    __ Title of article
    __ Full name(s), academic degrees, and institutional
       affiliations and status of author(s)
    __ Name of author to whom correspondence and galley proofs
       should be directed; include mailing address, business and
       home telephone numbers, and fax number
    __ Short title
__ Article proper (three copies, double-spaced)
__ Reference list (three copies, double-spaced, on a separate sheet)
__ Legends (three copies, double-spaced, on a separate sheet)
__ Tables (three copies, double-spaced, on a separate sheet)
__ Figures, properly labeled (three sets of glossy prints)
__ Written permission to reproduce previously published figures and
   consents to print photographs of identifiable likenesses of subjects

---

Note. From "Information for Authors," by P. R. Ebersole, 1993, *Geriatric Nursing, 14,* p. 118. Copyright 1993 by Mosby-Year Book Inc. Reprinted by permission of the publisher.

clude specific checklists for their journal along with their publishing guidelines. A careful final reading of the manuscript should be done, even though word processing spell and grammar checks have been conducted. Many journals now request both a copy of the manuscript on paper and on diskette.

A card or letter from the journal editor noting that the manuscript has been received should be received approximately 4 weeks after the manuscript has been sent. If a notification of receipt is not received, the first author should telephone the editor to determine if the manuscript has been received. Manuscripts do get lost, and early detection of the loss will prevent undue delays in review of the manuscript. The notification letter from the editor will usually inform authors about the length of the review process. Most nursing journals use a peer-review process in which the manuscript is sent to three or more reviewers.

Receiving the letter noting that a manuscript has been accepted for publications is a thrill to both the neophyte and the accomplished author. However, often some revisions are needed before the manuscript can be published. Authors are required to sign a form granting the publisher copyright privileges for the article. The editor will detail the issue of the journal in which the article will appear and when galley proofs can be expected. If an author knows that she or he will be absent during the time galley proofs are expected, arrangements should be made with the editor to have someone else proof them, as tight timelines exist for publishing an issue of a journal.

Authors receiving a "pink" slip (letter of rejection) should not be downhearted. Often the editor's letter contains feedback from the reviewers on revisions to be made that would make the manuscript acceptable for publication. Also, the editor may note that the particular topic is not one that is suitable for that journal. Thus, the author can seek publication in another journal.

Although the above discussion has largely focused on publishing in professional journals, APNs should also give attention to publishing in lay journals. Because nurses possess skills for speaking and interacting in a language that patients understand, these same skills can be used in developing manuscripts that will have wide public readership. Before submitting a manuscript, a sample of the type of article to be published could be sent to the health editor of the magazine. Nursing is receiving increasing media coverage, and many magazines may be receptive to feature articles by nurses.

PRESENTATIONS

Sharing of information with colleagues via presentations at professional meetings is another avenue that can be used to help advance the profession of nursing and establish a substantive knowledge base for nursing practice. Many opportunities at the local, regional, national, and international levels exist for the APN to share information with colleagues. "Calls" for abstracts for conferences are sent to members of professional organizations and are now often available on the Internet. The submitted abstracts are peer-reviewed, and presenters are notified. Typically, conferences offer opportunities for paper presentations and posters.

Abstracts

Writing an abstract appears to be a simple task. However, for many researchers, this task takes time because the background, problem statement, methodology, findings, and conclusions all have to be condensed and presented in a very few words, often 250 words or less. Thus, the author must carefully select the key points and then choose words that will enable the reviewers to understand the project. Too often, persons expend much space on one aspect of the project and neglect to describe all of the elements. Reviewers are then left to decide whether the missing elements were never addressed in the study or were omitted in the abstract. Having a colleague read the abstract before submitting it helps in achieving a "winning" abstract.

Fuller (1983) details important points for authors to consider when preparing abstracts. Elements to include in an abstract include the purpose, the design and methods, findings, and interpretation of findings or implications. The statement of purpose should incorporate the theoretical or conceptual framework upon which the study is based. This is important, as many studies in nursing have tended to be atheoretical and contribute only minimally to the development of nursing knowledge.

Poster

Posters have become a very popular method for sharing findings from research studies (McDaniel, Bach, & Poole, 1993). However, some persons still view presentations via a poster as being less prestigious than paper presentations. Sharing research via a poster is very rewarding, as it provides researchers with opportunities to engage in conversations with persons having a particular interest in their research. Such an opportunity is not available to persons making paper presentations.

Two methods are used for poster presentations: free-standing posters which are displayed on tables, and bulletin boards on which the materials are pinned. If the conference materials do not specify the type of display board, the presenter should obtain this information, as those specifications will dictate what the presenter needs to bring to the conference. For free-standing posters, the presenter needs to provide either a manufactured poster frame, or have pieces attached to poster board that can stand by itself. When a bulletin board is available, the presenter only needs to bring the poster piece(s) to attach.

Planning is critical to an effective poster presentation. Figure 13.1 depicts a sample layout for a poster presentation of research findings. Most often, three poster panels are used to present the content. If less table or bulletin board space is available, modifications will be needed. Key points to include in developing the poster are presented in Table 13.3.

Services of a graphics department are helpful in developing posters. However, computer graphics programs now allow tables and diagrams to be prepared in a less costly manner. Attractive colored backings can be used to mount pieces. Attaching velcro to the back of the mounted pieces allows them to be readily attached to cloth poster frames. Some presenters now generate the poster in one piece; this is handy, as it can be easily mounted for display. Whether the presenter is using a graphics department or constructing the poster by herself or himself, sufficient time in planning and developing the poster is needed. Lippman and Ponton (1989) recommend allowing 6 to 8 weeks for the process.

Presenting a poster is exciting. Wearing comfortable shoes is important, as the presenter may need to stand for a long time. Many poster presenters have abstracts available for the viewers. It is also helpful to have copies of instruments that were used in the study accessible for participants to review. Providing a sheet for participants to sign if they wish additional information about the project is appreciated.

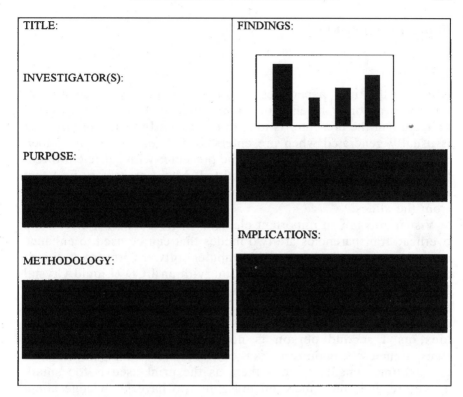

FIGURE 13.1   Sample layout for a poster presentation of research findings

TABLE 13.3   Key Points to Keep in Mind When Developing a Poster

Is the type readable from a distance?
   1-inch lettering can be read at 25 feet.
Does the layout provide for sufficient free space?
   Content should cover only about 50% of the space.
Can figures, tables, or pictures contribute to the clarity?
   These add variety and increase interest.
Are too many words used?
   Use of bullets and tables ease reading. Simplicity is important.
Are all the important points included?
   Having others critique the layout will help to identify points that have been omitted.
Do important points stand out?
   Spatial balance is important as is use of different colors and sizes of print.
Is the flow of content easily followed?
   Eye movement over the poster should be natural, left to right, and top to bottom.
   Arrows can be used to help the reader.
Does the poster have eye appeal?
   Selection of colors to match the background, use of contrasts, and avoidance of light
   colors add to the attractiveness of a poster.

Paper Presentation

Although the title "paper presentation" is frequently used when referring to an oral presentation of research, it does not necessarily indicate that the presenter is to read the paper. In fact, more interest is usually generated when presenters do not read the entire paper. Using a detailed outline provides the presenter with sufficient direction so that key content is not omitted. Many presenters find that placing key content on slides allows them the freedom to "talk" from the slides.

Visual aids are an important element of presentations. Slides and overhead transparencies are two modes that can be used to enhance oral presentations. Advances in computer software provide additional options. For example, Power Point with an LCD (Liquid Crystal Display) is being used by many presenters. Visual aids help to gain the audience's attention and identify the key points of the presentation. Using slides in presentations is much easier than transparencies, as a second person is not needed to take care of the transparencies. A major criticism of visual aids is that the audience is sometimes unable to read them as the print used is too small. Therefore, it is incumbent on presenters to have knowledge about the size of the room and about the size of the lettering needed for visual aids. Often presenters try to share too much information on slides and transparencies.

Selby, Tornquist, and Finerty (1989) noted that adequate preparation is key to a successful delivery. Knowledge about the length of time available for the presentation is needed before the person embarks on developing the paper. Fifteen- or 20-minute time frames are common time frames for papers at research conferences. Therefore, the presenter must select the key points to convey to the audience. Inclusion of content on the background and theoretical underpinnings are important, but prime attention should be given to the findings and conclusions. What are the main facts gained from doing the study and what are the implications, if any, that these have for practice and for future research? Audiences always welcome having time to ask questions at the conclusion of the presentation.

IMPLICATIONS FOR PREPARATION OF APNS

Educators need to ask themselves if opportunities are provided for APN students not only to be exposed to methods for professional communication, but to actively participate in these activities during their student days. Faculty members need to model these behaviors for students. Sharing information about research conferences or recent publications are ways to model this role. A more crucial point is to provide opportunities for students to publish or present their own research or evaluation findings. Encouragement from faculty is often needed for APN students to view their work as having value. Collaborating with students in writing an abstract for submission or developing a manuscript for publication will assist students in making communication an integral part of their roles as APNs. Nursing will be enriched when more APNs share their research, professional perspectives, and new practice models with the wider nursing community.

REFERENCES

American Psychological Association. (1994). *Publication manual of the American Psychological Association.* (4th ed.). Washington, DC: Author.

Barnum, B. S. (1995). *Writing and getting published.* New York: Springer Publishing Company.

Blancett, S. S. (1991). The ethics of writing and publishing. *Journal of Nursing Administration, 21*(5), 31–36.

Ebersole, P. R. (1993). Information for authors. *Geriatric Nursing, 14,* 118.

Fuller, E. (1983). Preparing an abstract for a nursing study. *Nursing Research, 32,* 316–317.

Herrin, J. (1989). Writing for a nursing journal. *Focus on Critical Care, 16,* 377–381.

Lippman, D. T., & Ponton, K. S. (1989). Designing a research poster with impact. *Western Journal of Nursing Research, 11,* 477–485.

McConnell, E. A. (1995). Journal and publishing characteristics for 42 nursing publications outside the United States. *Image: Journal of Nursing Scholarship, 27,* 225–229.

McDaniel, R. W., Bach, C. A., & Poole, M. J. (1993). Poster update: getting their attention. *Nursing Research, 42,* 302–304.

Midwest Nursing Research Society. (1996). *Guidelines for scientific integrity.* Glenview, IL: Author.

Plawecki, H. M., & Plawecki, J. A. (1998). Writing of publication: Understanding the process. *Journal of Holistic Nursing, 16*(1), 23–32.

Robinson, D., Collins, M., & Monkman, J. (1997). A practice guide to writing for publication. *Nurse Researcher, 5*(1), 53–64.

Ryden, M. (1998). Active listening. In M. Snyder & R. Lindquist (Eds.), *Complementary/Alternative therapies in nursing* (3rd ed., pp. 169–180). New York: Springer Publishing Company.

Scott, D. H. (1989). *Secrets of successful writing.* San Francisco: Reference Software International.

Selby, M. L., Tornquist, E. M., & Finerty, E. J. (1989). How to present your research. *Nursing Outlook, 37,* 172–175.

Servodidio, C. A. (1998). Writing Tips for Authors. *Insight, 23*(1), 24–27.

Sheridan, D. R., & Dowdney, D. L. (1997). *How to write and publish articles in nursing, 2nd edition.* New York: Springer Publishing Company.

Stevens, K. R. (1986). Authorship: Yours, mine, or ours? *Image: Journal of Nursing Scholarship, 18,* 151–154.

Styles, M. M. (1978). Why publish? *Image, 10*(2), 28–32.

Swanson, E. A., McCloskey, J. C., & Bodensteiner, A. (1991). *Image: Journal of Nursing Scholarship, 23,* 33–38.

Tucker-Allen, S. (1997). The publication process: Steps to success. *ABNF Journal, 8*(3), 58–63.

Zorn, C. R., Smith, M. C., & Werley, H. H. (1991). Watch your language. *Nursing Outlook, 39,* 183–185.

Chapter 14

CLIENT ADVOCACY

Margot L. Nelson, PhD, RN, CS

The role of advocate for the patient or client[1] and the implementation of advocacy as an intervention have been acclaimed moral imperatives, integral to the profession and practice of nursing. Legitimate questions have been raised, however, about the authenticity with which nurses are able to advocate for clients in contexts which also obligate nurses to advocate for health systems and health care dollars. Nurses in advanced practice roles are able to negotiate these conflicting expectations by virtue of their expertise, relative autonomy of practice, engagement in interdisciplinary decision-making, and commitment to the health of communities.

DEFINITIONS

A definition which synthesizes much of the theory and research relative to nurse advocacy is that it is a "way of being in relationship with a

---

[1]The terms "client" and "patient" are used interchangeably throughout this chapter to refer to a recipient of health care in general and nursing care in particular.

patient/client, a way of being which respects and promotes the uniqueness of the (client) as a total human being in the context of his/her health experience" (Nelson, 1992, p. 263). It is a characteristic of the nurse as a person, not just what he or she does. In an advocacy role, the nurse assists individuals to find meaning in their living or dying; and Curtin (1979) emphasizes that it is the patient's experience, meaning and values that are of concern—not the experience, meaning, and values of the nurse or anyone else. Watson (1989) refers to advocacy as an outgrowth of caring, that foundational aspect of nursing in which an authentic and intimate connection occurs between nurse and patient, enabling the patient to find his/her "own voice" (p. 53).

Advocacy is viewed by some nurse authors (Curtin, 1979; Gadow, 1980a) as an essential component of the philosophical basis for nursing. Curtin describes advocacy as closely associated with the nurse-patient relationship, rooted in a shared humanity and human rights (freedom, respect, and integrity). Curtin's emphasis on the nurse-patient relationship is supported by findings of a recent qualitative study exploring nurses' views of patient advocacy (Chafey, Rhea, Shannon, & Spencer, 1998) in which British nurses identified relational qualities as more essential to nurse advocacy than accountability and ethics.

Gadow (1980a, 1980b, 1989, 1990) is the most frequently quoted source for the philosophical underpinnings of advocacy in nursing. Gadow promotes existential advocacy in nursing, whereby patients are enabled to exercise self-determination in the context of their unique personal meanings and health experiences. Authentically exercising freedom of self-determination, according to Gadow, means reaching decisions that are truly one's own and that reflect what one values and believes important about oneself and the world.

Kavanagh (1994) suggests cultural congruence as an additional dimension for advocacy. If a nurse engages in culturally congruent advocacy, she or he enables the client to maintain the integrity of his or her own perspectives and ways of being. To do this, the nurse must make a conscious effort not to impose the values of the dominant culture on persons and groups from other cultures.

Joel (1998) has included advocacy as one of the integral roles for advanced practice nurses, along with case management, triage, and staff development. Joel discusses these roles in conjunction with the increasingly complex health status of patients and the changing context of health care. Clinical nurse specialists themselves ranked client and family advocacy as their most frequent direct caregiving activity in a survey conducted by McMillan, Heusinkveld & Spray (1995).

EVOLUTION OF THE ADVOCACY ROLE IN NURSING

A review of the historical development of advocacy provides a fuller understanding of advocacy. In keeping with the evolution of professional nursing, advocacy has progressed from interceding for a client to acting as guardian of client rights to promoting autonomy and free choice for all health care consumers. It continues to evolve with the shift from a paradigm of illness to a paradigm encompassing health as the focus of health care, the community as the primary site for health care delivery, and the advanced practice nurse as a primary health care provider. The stages of development have been discussed thoroughly elsewhere (Nelson, 1988; Nelson, 1998). The most recent version of advocacy emphasizes the client's rights and autonomy in decision making as the unconditional first priorities.

DEBATES ABOUT THE CONGRUENCE OF ADVOCACY WITH NURSING

Proponents frequently use Gadow's (1980a) philosophical articulation as the basis for their support of advocacy in nursing. Gadow described the nurse as an existential advocate, responding to individuals' needs to authentically exercise their freedom of self-determination:

> The nurse advocate helps persons become clear about what it is they want to do, by helping them discern and clarify their values in the situation and only on the basis of that self-examination, to reach decisions, which express their reaffirmed, perhaps recreated, complex of values. (p. 85)

Authors since then have supported nurses as optimally positioned for this role by virtue of

1) the unique, intimate and continuous relationship nurses have with patients and families,
2) the opportunity such proximity provides for knowledge of patients' meanings, values, and preferences,

3) specialized educational preparation of nurses for a negotiator role, and

4) the nurses' in-between location—between clients and other providers, between clients and the health care system, and between clients and families.

These supportive arguments are particularly relevant for nurses in advanced practice roles.

Love (1995) calls for advanced practice nurses to assume the role of client advocate with respect to end-of-life decisions, asserting that even mentally competent clients and their families may not be able to verbalize their questions, needs, and preferences because of intimidation or the perception that health care providers don't have time to listen. She further argues that other elements may interfere with decision-making: fear, depression, confusion, and the enormous stress imposed by health and illness experiences. Patients in a weakened state are at risk of being manipulated or coerced by others, or may simply not have the energy to maintain a position which is not supported by their primary care providers or their families.

There are, nevertheless, cogent arguments against the assumption of a client advocacy role by nurses. Mallik (1997) contrasts nursing advocacy with legal advocacy. When an attorney enters into an advocacy agreement (legal advocacy) with a client, there is a formal contract between them. In nursing advocacy, the nurse claims the role of advocate on the basis of his or her professional way of being, without regard to clients' expectations or desires that nurses serve as their advocates. Furthermore, clients may be subtly coerced to follow the nurse's preferences by their dependence on nurses for care and information (Mackereth, 1995), raising ethical questions about the trust they can place in nurses as their advocates.

Client powerlessness (Namerow, 1982; Webb, 1987; Winslow, 1984) and vulnerability (Copp, 1986; Mallik, 1997) are frequently used to justify the need for nurse advocacy. But doubts have been raised regarding nurses' autonomy in health care (Gaylord & Grace, 1995) and whether one relatively powerless group (nurses) can effectively represent another (Mallik, 1997). Although a real proponent of advocacy in nursing, Curtin (1983) has questioned the realism with which nurse advocates have been portrayed in the literature: "as a combination lawyer-theologian-psychologist-family counselor and dragon slayer wrapped up in a white uniform" (p. 9). Not only have the white uniforms become less representative of nurses, particularly those in advanced practice, but the call to more realistic expectations should be heeded.

Recent research findings raise questions of the degree to which nurses can navigate the tensions created by hierarchical structures in the health care system, responsibilities to employers and physicians, and commitments to clients. In a 1987 study by Savage, Cullen, Kirchhoff, Pugh, and Forman, nurses' ethical decision making was found to be influenced more by their perceptions of what others expected of them than by their own moral reasoning. In another study of nurses' decision making (Millette, 1993), two-thirds of 222 practicing nurses indicated a preference for client advocacy versus institution and physician advocacy. But only a small number selected the actions of a client advocate as the best responses to case presentations. Choices reflected greater concern for the institution than for the client, particularly by nurse managers and nurses practicing in acute care settings.

In summary, the debate continues about whether nurses can realistically assume the role of client advocate, particularly in light of the nurse as instigator of the role and the nurse's divided loyalties. There is no doubt that in some circumstances the nurse is cast as a "double agent," attempting to represent both patient and physician, more than one patient, or patient and health care institution (Nelson, 1988). Surmounting the barriers which exist in many settings calls advanced practice nurses to solidly reclaim their commitments to nursing and the health of communities, daring to "imagine transformative possibilities" and to "run with the wolves" (Rafael, 1998, p. 41).

APPLICATION OF ADVOCACY TO ADVANCED NURSING PRACTICE

Johnson (1993) has documented the practice of advocacy by advanced practice nurses in primary care settings, contrasting the nurses' paradigm with that of their medical counterparts. The apparent medical ideology viewed people as biologic systems with clear separation of mind and body, while the nursing view of the person was more holistic (valuing the mind, body and spirit connections) and attuned to the "lifeworld" or personal experience of the client. This nursing perspective was reflected in greater attention to establishing relationships with clients, sharing a language, considering the context of the clients' "lifeworlds", and proposing more personalized responses to health concerns. Brykczynski (1993) describes these findings as capturing the "elusive process of care" (p.159), which undergirds the implementation of advocacy.

Types of Advocacy

A typology of advocacy in nursing has been proposed by Nelson (1992), synthesizing frameworks of Curtin (1979) and Fowler (1989). Five forms of advocacy are described: legal advocacy, moral-ethical advocacy, substitutive advocacy, political advocacy, and spiritual advocacy. The common goal of all these types of advocacy is to facilitate the client's exercise of rights to self-determination related to health and to promote decision making congruent with who the person is, what he/she values, and the level of self-determination possible at a given point in time. Snowball (1996) refers to these specific and individual responses to immediate needs or risks in a clinical situation as reactive advocacy. Proactive advocacy, by contrast, addresses the bigger picture of health care through sharing of information, influencing health policy, and incorporating the voices of clients into the planning of health care, all elements of advanced nursing practice. Advocacy for nursing and advocacy for the community's health have therefore been added to Nelson's earlier typology. See Table 14.1.

Legal advocacy

Clients' legal rights form the basis for legal advocacy, including rights to be informed, to accept or refuse treatment, and to be protected from incompetent, illegal, or unethical practices. Actions empowering patients in their interaction with the health care system fit within this model of advocacy.

Segesten (1993) reported that the most common impetus for advocacy, based on the narrative accounts of expert nurses, involves patients' rights to decide for themselves and highlight the criteria for informed consent: adequate information to make rational decisions, mental competence on the part of the decision maker, and uncoerced, freely given consent (Grodin, Kaminov, & Sassower, 1986). Informed consent means that available alternatives have been presented and understood, including a discussion of risks and probability of success for each alternative.

TABLE 14.1 Types of Advocacy for Advanced Practice Nurses

Type	Role of the Advocate	Underpinnings
Legal Advocacy	Guardian of client rights	Individual, group, and community rights (e. g. to informed consent, refusal of treatment, accessibility to competent care, and privacy)
Moral-ethical advocacy	Sustainer of client values	Awareness of values and congruent decision making
Substitutive advocacy	Supporter of client voice and best interests	Preservation of rights for persons who are unable to speak for themselves
Political advocacy	Champion of social justice	Equal access to nursing and health care
Spiritual advocacy	Existential and authentic presence	Spiritual comfort and counsel in the quest for meaning
Advocate for nursing	Facilitator of professional growth	Demonstration of and contribution to the excellence of nursing
Advocate for the community's health	Promoter of the community's health	Facilitating health of population aggregates

Note. Adapted from "Advocacy," by M. L. Nelson, in M. Snyder and R. Lindquist (Eds.), *Complementary/Alternative therapies in Nursing* (3rd ed., p. 341), 1998, New York: Springer Publishing Company. Copyright 1998 by Springer Publishing Company. Adapted with permission.

Foss (Nelson, 1993c), a clinical nurse specialist, has described situations in which "patients and families may not be getting the answers they need because they . . . don't know the right questions to ask." Foss depicts her role as helping people articulate these questions and serving as interpreter when other providers use complex medical terms with a family that needs to have things explained more simply. Advocacy by advanced practice nurses may take the form of ascertaining a client's competence to understand, being the primary purveyor of information, updating or clarifying information provided by another professional, and evaluating the client's and family's understanding.

Other legal rights which the nurse is obliged to protect are the right to privacy, the right to refuse procedures or providers, and the freedom to leave an institution which is providing care. Privacy is protected by sharing personal information about clients only in the context of facilitating care provision and by expecting other health care providers to treat such information with the same respect. Clients and families, perceiving the power differential between themselves and health care providers, are often unaware of the right to refuse medications, tests, procedures, treatments, or care providers. It is imperative, therefore, that the nurse advocate make these rights known.

The bottom line in legal advocacy is that rights belong to the patient, which means that he or she also has the right not to exercise those rights. It means, further, that patient choices must be accepted and support of the patient continued, even when the nurse disagrees with the choices.

Moral-ethical advocacy

Moral-ethical advocacy is based upon honoring patient values and facilitating decision making congruent with those values. It requires that the patient desire self-determination and have the ability to participate in values exploration and decision making. In this type of advocacy, every encounter is viewed through a lens of respect for the uniqueness of the person and his/her situation and time. The intent of the nurse is to preserve or clarify patient values and assure autonomy in decision making, providing the professional assistance desired by the client. Nurses often serve as the communication link among members of the health team, the patient, and the family (Copp, 1986) and act as "culture brokers" (Jezewski, 1993), bridging the gaps in cultural meaning and understanding between at least two cultures: the culture of the client and that of the health care system.

A prerequisite for this type of advocacy is an existential relationship between nurse and client, described by Gadow (1980b) as being attuned to each other, expressing their wholeness and uniqueness in a clarification and sharing of values. Objections have occasionally been raised to the nurse's authentic sharing of personal views or even to pursuing clarification of patient values on the grounds that this may undermine the patient's decisional autonomy (Kohnke, 1982). The nurse advocate walks a fine line between "clarification" and "subtle manipulation" (p. 29). It is critical, therefore, to assure that the emphasis is upon the client's values and desires.

The advanced practice nurse is frequently in a position to help individual clients, families, and groups clarify their values or to counsel other nurses toward fulfilling this role. Miller (Nelson, 1993b), a geriatric clinical specialist, has described her role in supporting clients to clarify their values and desired outcomes, "letting them know it's okay for them to decide or even to disagree with their doctor." Another useful intervention is to invite and encourage clients of any age or condition to consider their values related to life, health, and death prior to situations of crisis or threat to life (Omery & Caswell, 1989). Discussions might include the option of an advanced directive (living will or durable power of attorney for health care) to identify the kinds of medical intervention one would desire or wish to refuse under potentially life-threatening circumstances, thus allowing clients to exercise control over their destinies "before-the-fact" (Grady, 1989).

Corcoran (1988) cautions that in all decisional support interventions the nurse must be qualified to provide accurate information. This means he or she must possess appropriate knowledge, communication skills, and rapport with the client. The advanced nurse clinician is an appropriate advocate by virtue of his or her expertise in knowledge and communication.

Substitutive advocacy

Substitutive advocacy is relevant when the patient is unable to express his or her own wishes and an identified proxy decision-maker is unavailable to speak on his/her behalf. The underlying principle is that every person has the ultimate right to speak for him/herself, so advocacy as a substitute for the client's own decision making is not something to be embarked upon lightly.

In instances where mental incapacity or lack of responsiveness clearly precludes the client's self-expression, it is important that someone serve as a voice for his or her preferences. This is obviously much easier when discussions with that person have previously occurred (Benner, 1981; Wolff, 1992).

Foss (Nelson, 1993c), a pulmonary clinical specialist, describes "translating (clients') issues and points of view to other players (on the health care team)." This translation may be appropriate for mentally competent as well as incompetent patients in some circumstances—for example, helping family members and other care providers understand how shortness of breath and anxiety affect the life experience of a person with chronic lung disease.

Efforts to change traditional patterns of care provision may also be viewed as a kind of substitutive advocacy. For example, some of the acute care practices which were routine early in the AIDS epidemic have been modified to become less restrictive. In many settings where there was a traditional policy of "family-only" visiting and involvement in decision making, the client is now asked to identify those who should be involved.

Substitutive advocacy, although not a desirable first option, is sometimes necessary because of circumstances prohibiting patients from acting on their own behalf. The advanced practice nurse may be in a prime position to serve as a proxy voice. With the growth in numbers of people with chronic health conditions and increased care provision in the community (Hicks, Stallmeyer, & Coleman, 1992), this form of advocacy has even broader application to self-and family care and forming networks across health care settings and providers.

Political advocacy

Also referred to as the "champion of social justice" role, political advocacy is based on the ethic of justice (universal access to adequate nursing and health care). It calls for nurses to actively strive for change on behalf of individuals, groups, and society as a whole so that inequities and inconsistencies are identified and corrected. This form of advocacy frequently requires action at a policy and legislative level. Nursing history is rich with nurse role models in this arena, including Florence Nightingale; Lavinia Dock, who addressed the problem of venereal disease through writing and public health actions; and Margaret Sanger, who provided leadership to meet women's health needs and to educate the public about birth control options.

Today political advocacy is more expedient through professional organizations than individual efforts in order to influence change in such areas as health care quality and access. As an example, the American Nurses Association (ANA) is attempting to influence change in health care accessibility and financing as well as availability of long-term care facilities, homes, and apartments for persons with AIDS and other chronic illnesses. Sohier (1992) calls nurses to respond to even broader issues such as hunger, poverty, homelessness, and illiteracy on a global level.

Collectively, nurses comprise a large voting block and a potentially powerful lobby. Advanced practice nurses are in positions to model and encourage other nurses to take advantage of their potential power (e.g., supporting nurse membership on health policy-making boards and councils). Because of their community visibility through practice across health care settings, the voices of advanced practice nurses are more readily heard and respected in addressing health issues of groups and communities.

Spiritual advocacy

This type of advocacy is based upon individual rights to spiritual comfort and access to clergy of choice. Since the search for meaning is both an ethical and a spiritual task, spiritual advocacy could be considered a subcategory of moral-ethical advocacy. Gadow (1980a) references spiritual advocacy when she discusses the nurse's interaction with the patient to determine the unique personal meaning that a health experience has for that individual. Through advocacy, nurses communicate sensitivity to personal hopes and values and create an atmosphere of caring and a sense of the possible. In addition to collaborating with and referring clients to clergy and counselors, nurses implement spiritual advocacy by being fully present and open to participate with and enter the "lifeworld" (Johnson, 1993) of patients in their search for meaning.

Advocacy for nursing

Just as client powerlessness signals a need for advocacy, Schmieding (1993) suggests that a perceived powerlessness in nurse colleagues provides an opportunity for advocacy. A unique dimension of advocacy for the advanced practice nurse is that of facilitating professional growth for other nurses and contributing to the evolution of nursing as a discipline. The form this kind of advocacy takes naturally depends on the setting of practice and the advanced clinician's role in that setting.

Both professional development for individual nurses and growth of the discipline may be fostered by the advanced clinician's leadership. The infusion of current research and literature into practice decisions and patient care is one way in which individual and group nursing practice may be enriched (Nelson, 1993a). The advanced practice nurse may also provide educational opportunities for mid-level practitioners as well as one-to-one "coaching" interactions stimulating critical thinking and accountability (Nelson, 1993a; 1993b; 1993c). Research and publishing represent formal avenues for contributing to knowledge development in the discipline. Involvement in education through schools of nursing allows for advocacy through upholding standards for new nurses entering into the profession (Snowball, 1996).

The advanced practice nurse may serve as a resource, consultant, mediator, mentor, or role model for other nurses. Because advanced practice nurses often have broader visibility, they have the opportunity to demonstrate the expertise and excellence of nursing to clients, members of other health care disciplines, and the community.

Advocacy for the community's health

Facilitating the health of population aggregates, while it is an assumed role for all professional nurses, is a defining characteristic of advanced nursing practice. The community's health is a pivotal concern for advanced practice nurses as they provide care in multiple settings and in the transitions between settings. Critical components of community-focused nursing include community assessments, identification of high-risk individuals, families, and groups in the community, and evaluation of the appropriateness of health policies, accessibility of health services, and environmental factors in the community. An additional role is assuring the presence of the community's (client's) voice in describing its own health and establishing priorities in health planning (Bunkers, Nelson, Leuning, Crane, & Josephson, in press).

FUTURE DEVELOPMENTS

Advocacy fits well with the evolution of advanced nursing practice. The complexity and transitional status of the health care system pose challenges to advocacy roles, but also underscore the need to protect the rights of health care consumers and assure that their voices are heard. In order to refine and expand the concept and practice of advocacy in nursing, attention needs to be given to measurement of its effectiveness and to further research.

Measurement of Effectiveness

Since advocacy includes a significant ethical dimension, ethical principles can serve as standards for evaluation. For example, if one uses nonmaleficence (the principle of causing no harm) as a guide, one of the most basic expected outcomes of advocacy is that the client not be hurt by advocacy interventions. If beneficence serves as a standard, advocacy should in some way promote the well-being of the client. With autonomy as a guiding principle, the client's self-determination must be included as a measure of effectiveness. If justice is a priority, a measure of fairness or equity in distributing health resources is in order. Fidelity suggests that we evaluate fulfillment of obligations, such as provision of care until a satisfactory alternative is found, following through with commitments, and honoring privacy and confidentiality.

The framework for advocacy illustrated in Table 14.1 also provides guidelines for posing evaluative questions about whether advocacy has been effective. Each form of advocacy provides somewhat different guidelines and questions. For legal advocacy, the client's legal rights must be upheld, and he or she must be able to verbalize understanding of those rights and resources available to assist with their protection. Specific rights and related questions are:

1. *Informed consent.* Has the client been provided the desired information about treatment or other health-related alternatives? Is he or she competent to give consent or been provided the opportunity to identify a proxy decisionmaker? Barring this, have earnest attempts been made to determine the substance of previously written or verbalized advanced directives? Does the client feel free to make choices without penalty or pressure from health care providers?
2. *Acceptance or refusal.* Can the client verbalize understanding of his or her right to refuse treatment or a specific health care provider? Is there opportunity for the client to express doubt or ambivalence and to ask questions?
3. *Protection from incompetent or unethical practices.* Are quality assurance measures in place to assure client safety and the competence of health care providers? Are procedures in place (and utilized) to intervene when there are threats to client safety or rights? Does the client know whom to contact with concerns about quality of care?

4. *Privacy and confidentiality.* Is access to client information treated in a privileged manner, assuring that details are shared only in the context of concern for the client and provision of health care? Is permission sought from the client prior to sharing confidential information?

For moral-ethical advocacy, the nurse-client relationship and the client's opportunity to be authentic with himself and a caring other are the focus of evaluation. Has the client been given the opportunity to explore personal values that are relevant to the present health situation? Have opportunities been provided for considering advanced directives regarding future life, health, and death decisions? Does the client have the degree of much control over health planning that he or she desires?

For substitutive advocacy, the major concern is that the best interests of the client are protected when he or she is unable to participate actively in the planning process. Have attempts been made to determine what wishes the client would express if he/she were able? Have the safety and dignity of the client been maintained? Have significant others been allowed and assisted to participate in care and decision making? Do client perspectives inform community health planning processes?

For political advocacy, nurses need to participate individually and collectively in actions to promote such goals as a healthy environment and accessible and affordable health care for all. Are nurses visible in community, state, regional, and national organizations and agencies that promote societal awareness of threats to health, seek health-related policy and legislative changes, and strive for resolution of economic and health care inequities? Are the voices of clients heard?

For spiritual advocacy, clients must be supported as they search for meaning in their health experiences, living, and dying. Is the nurse open and present with the client in such a way that meaningful interchange about spiritual concerns can occur? Is there an attitude of caring and hope on the part of the nurse? Are clients' unique personal meanings sought and respected? Are opportunities provided for client contact with the clergy of choice? Has communication been maintained despite the client's level of response?

In advocacy for nursing, a critical concern is the direction of professional growth and the visibility of nursing in the community. How do members of other health care disciplines and the community perceive the contribution of nursing to the health of the community? Do individual nurses' career trajectories reflect an increasing depth of knowledge, expertise, and professional commitment? Are standards of excellence upheld in the selection, progression, and graduation of nurses from educational programs?

In advocacy for the community's health, many specific indicators may be utilized to evaluate aspects of the community's health, from infant mortality rates, to sexual practices of various age groups, tobacco use, and the incidence of HIV infection and cancer. Pivotal questions must relate to the community's appraisal of its own health. How do members of the community and of specific population groups view their health? Are these voices represented in community health decision making arenas?

Some of these questions can be answered through information in clients' health records, others subjectively by the clients themselves or by the nurse. Others, such as those pertaining to spiritual advocacy, can only be intuited by an observer or perhaps only by the participants in a nurse-client relationship. Still others require a more rigorous evaluation of the profession and the community.

Research Directions

There has been little research related to advocacy in nursing, with the exception of some early attempts to identify role priorities for physicians and nurses in specific settings and Murphy's (1983) and Millette's (1993) study of nurses' decision making according to advocacy preferences. Particularly in advanced nursing practice, research is needed to refine the concept, explicate the ways in which advocacy can be operationalized, and document client outcomes. A few of the relevant questions which might be asked are these:

1. To what extent do nurses perceive themselves as advocates and for whom (clients, families, communities, institutions, or physicians)?
2. What are the needs for advocacy in specific population groups?
3. To what extent do clients expect and desire advanced practice nurses to serve as their advocates? How are specific advocacy interventions received?
4. How do advocacy behaviors on the part of the nurse affect the congruence between clients' values and their health-related decisions? other potential outcomes?
5. What is the experience of the advanced practice nurse as advocate? How is this experienced by the client?

Nursing's paradigm entails a basic ethical commitment to the rights and well-being of patients (American Nurses Association, 1985) and to understanding human health experiences through the eyes of those who live them (Newman, Sime, & Corcoran-Perry, 1991). These professional underpinnings make advocacy for the client a first priority, even in situations where fulfilling this priority may need to be delegated to another person in order for the client's cause to be most fairly represented. It is also congruent with some of the major nursing theories. Advocacy is present in what Watson (1988) describes as a transpersonal caring relationship, encompassing "high regard for the whole person and their being-in-the-world" (p. 63) and basic concern for human dignity. It is also reflected in Parse's (1992) description of the process of becoming as one in which individuals freely choose personal meaning and in the emphasis Parse places on quality of life from the individual's own perspective. Newman's theory of health as expanding consciousness (1994) reflects advocacy through honoring persons' meaning as they are revealed in unfolding patterns. These theories, and perhaps others, can therefore be used as a foundation for research and for practice models related to advocacy in nursing. It is important that advanced practice nurses attend to the barriers and possible pitfalls as well as the obligations to advocacy in light of their own professional values and commitments.

REFERENCES

American Nurses Association. (1985). *Code for nurses with interpretive statements.* Kansas City, MO: American Nurses Association.

Benner, P. (1981). "Commentary." In B. DeCoste (Ed.), *The many faces of advocacy* (p. 82). *American Journal of Nursing, 81,* 80–82.

Brykzynski, K. A. (1993). Response to "Nurse Practitioner-Patient Discourse: Uncovering the voice of nursing in primary care practice. " *Scholarly Inquiry for Nursing Practice, 7,* 159–163.

Bunkers, S. S., Nelson, M. L., Leuning, C., Crane, J., & Josephson, D. (In press). The Health Action Model: Academia's partnership with the community. In E. L. Cohen & V. DeBack (Eds.), *The outcomes mandate: Case management in health care today* (pp. 92–100). St. Louis: Mosby.

Chafey, K., Rhea, M., Shannon, A. M., & Spencer, S. (1998). Characterizations of advocacy by practicing nurses. *Journal of Professional Nursing, 14,* 43–52.

Copp, L. A. (1986). The nurse as advocate for vulnerable persons. *Journal of Advanced Nursing, 11,* 255–263.

Copp, L. A. (1993). Response to "Patient advocacy: An important part of the daily work of the expert nurse. " *Scholarly Inquiry for Nursing Practice, 7,* 137–140.

Corcoran, S. (1988). Toward operationalizing an advocacy role. *Journal of Professional Nursing, 4,* 242–248.

Curtin, L. L. (1979). The nurse as advocate: A philosophical foundation for nursing. *Nursing Science, 1,* 1–10.

Fowler, M. D. M. (1989). Social advocacy. *Heart & Lung, 18,* 97–99.

Gadow, S. (1980a). Existential advocacy: Philosophical foundation of nursing. In S. F. Spicker & S. Gadow (Eds.), *Nursing, images and ideals: Opening dialogue with the humanities* (pp 79–89). New York: Springer Publishing Company.

Gadow, S. (1980b). A model for ethical decision making. *Oncology Nursing Forum, 7,* 44–47.

Gadow, S. (1989). Clinical subjectivity: advocacy with silent patients. *Nursing Clinics of North America, 24,* 535–541.

Gadow, S. (1990). Existential advocacy: philosophical foundations of nursing. In T. Pence & J. Cantrell (Eds.), *Ethics in nursing: An anthology* (pp. 41–52). New York: National League for Nursing.

Gaylord, N., & Grace, P. (1995). Nursing advocacy: An ethic of practice. *Nursing Ethics, 2,* 11–18.

Grady, C. (1989). Ethical issues in providing nursing care to human immunodeficiency virus-infected populations. *Journal of Advanced Nursing, 14,* 513–514.

Grodin, M., Kaminov, P., & Sassower, R. (1986). Ethical issues in AIDS research. *Quarterly Review Bulletin, 10,* 347–352.

Hicks, L., Stallmeyer, J. M., & Coleman, J. R. (1992). Nursing challenges in managed care. *Nursing Economic$, 10,* 265–276.

Jezewski, M. A. (1993). Culture brokering as a model for advocacy. *Nursing & Health Care, 14,* 78–85.

Joel, L. A. (1998). Advanced practice nursing in the current sociopolitical environment. In C. M. Sheehy, & M. C. McCarthy (Eds.), *Advanced practice nursing: Emphasizing common roles* (pp. 47–67). Philadelphia: F. A. Davis.

Johnson, R. (1993). Nurse-practitioner-patient discourse: Uncovering the voice of nursing in primary care practice. *Scholarly Inquiry for Nursing Practice, 7,* 143–157.

Kavanagh, K. H. (1994). Trancultural nursing: Facing the challenges of advocacy and diversity/universality. *Journal of Transcultural Nursing, 5,* 4–13.

Kohnke, M. F. (1982). *Advocacy: Risk and Reality.* St. Louis: Mosby.

Love, M. B. (1995). Patient advocacy at the end of life. *Nursing Ethics, 2,* 3–9.

Mackereth, P. A. (1995). HIV and homophobia: nurses as advocates. *Journal of Advanced Nursing, 22,* 670–676.

Mallik, M. (1997). Advocacy in nursing: A review of the literature. *Journal of Advanced Nursing, 25,* 130–138.

McMillan, S. C., Heusinkveldt, K. B., & Spray, J. (1995). Advanced practice in oncology nursing: A role delineation study. *Oncology Nursing Forum, 22,* 41–50.

Millette, B. E. (1993). Client advocacy and the moral orientation of nurses. *Western Journal of Nursing Research, 15,* 607.

Murphy, C. P. (1983). Models of the nurse-patient relationship. In C. P. Murphy & H. Hunter (Eds.), *Ethical Problems in the Nurse-Patient Relationship* (pp. 8–24). New York: Allyn & Bacon.

Namerow, M. J. (1982). Integrating advocacy into the gerontological nursing major. *Journal of Gerontological Nursing, 8,* 149–151.

Nelson, M. L. (1988). Advocacy in nursing. *Nursing Outlook, 36,* 136–141.

Nelson, M. L. (1992). Advocacy. In M. Snyder (Ed.), *Independent nursing interventions* (pp. 262–273). Albany: Delmar Publishers.

Nelson, M. L. (1993c). [Unpublished interview with Ann Mulkey, family nurse practitioner]. Unpublished raw data.

Nelson, M. L. (1993b). [Unpublished interview with Doreen S. Miller, geriatric clinical specialist]. Unpublsihed raw data.

Nelson, M. L. (1993c). [Unpublished interview with Nancy Foss, pulmonary clinical nurse specialist]. Unpublished raw data.

Nelson, M. L. (1998). Advocacy. In M. Snyder, & R. Lindquist, (Eds.), *Complementary/Alternative therapies in nursing 3rd ed,* pp. 337–352. New York: Springer Publishing Company.

Newman, M. A., Sime, A. M., & Corcoran-Perry, S. A. (1991). The focus of the discipline of nursing. *Advances in Nursing Science, 14,* 1–6.

Newman, M. A. (1994). *Health as expanding consciousness (2nd ed.).* New York: National League for Nursing.

Omery, A., & Caswell, D. (1989). Ethical perspectives. *Critical Care Nursing Clinics of North America, 1,* 165–173.

Parse, R. R. (1992). Human becoming: Parse's theory of nursing. *Nursing Science Quarterly, 5,* 35–42.

Rafael, A. R. F. (1998). Nurses who run with the wolves: The power and caring dialectic revisited. *Advances in Nursing Science, 21,* 29–42.

Savage, T. A., Cullen, D. L., Kirchhoff, K. T., Pugh, E. J., & Forman, M. D. (1987). Nurses' responses to do-not-resuscitate orders in the neonatal intensive care unit. *Nursing Research, 36,* 370–373.

Schmieding, N. J. (1993). Nurse empowerment through context, structure, and process. *Journal of Professional Nursing, 9,* 239–245.

Segesten, K. (1993). Patient advocacy: An important part of the daily work of the expert nurse. *Scholarly Inquiry for Nursing, 7,*129–135.

Snowball, J. (1996). Asking nurses about advocating for patients: "Reactive" and "proactive" accounts. *Journal of Advanced Nursing, 24,* 67–75.

Sohier, R. (1992). Feminism and nursing knowledge: The power of the weak. *Nursing Outlook, 40,* 62–66, 93.

Watson, J. (1989). Transformative thinking and a caring curriculum. In E. O.

Bevis, & J. Watson, J. (Eds.), *Toward a caring curriculum: A new pedagogy for nursing*. New York: National League for Nursing.

Watson, J. (1988). *Nursing: Human science and human care, a theory of nursing*. New York: National League for Nursing.

Watson, J. (1992). Response to "Caring, virtue theory, and a foundation for nursing ethics. " *Scholarly Inquiry for Nursing Practice, 6,* 169–171.

Webb, C. (1987). Speaking up for advocacy. *Nursing Times, 83,* 33–35.

Winslow, G. R. (1984). From loyalty to advocacy: A new metaphor for nursing. *Hastings Center Report, 14,* 32–40.

Wolff, T. L. (1992). The community health nurse as advocate. *Home Healthcare Nurse, 10,* 14–17, 78–79.

Chapter 15

ETHICAL ISSUES IN ADVANCED PRACTICE NURSING

M. Cecilia Wendler, RN, MA, CCRN

Ethical dilemmas are ubiquitous in nursing practice (Cassidy & Oddi, 1988; O'Neil, 1991; Wagner & Ronen, 1996). Many nurses are not prepared to make ethical decisions (Catalano, 1991, 1997) and lack and understanding of the philosophical foundations which underpin these decisions (Aroskar, 1986; O'Neil, 1991; Smith, 1996). Further, nurses historically have often not been successful in influencing ethical decisions and have exhibited biases such as ethnocentrism within the nurse-patient relationship (Greipp, 1995; Holly & Lyons, 1993). In the integrated roles of educator, leader, and consultant. the advanced practice nurse is uniquely prepared and positioned to become actively involved in facilitating and influencing ethical decision making (Clochesy, Daly, Idemota, Steel, & Fitzpatric, 1994; Harris, 1997; Holly & Lyons, 1993; Kachoyeanos & Zollo, 1995; Snyder & Yen, 1995).

A consciously chosen ethical framework appropriately applied may facilitate the ethical power of individuals and staffs by providing an assistive template for data-gathering that supports reflective thinking (Aroskar, 1986; Gadow, 1983; Holly & Lyons, 1993). In this chapter, an overview of current ethical thinking in nursing and a description and application of an ethical-decision making framework will be provided.

BACKGROUND

Ethics is a branch of theology and philosophy which is concerned with what is right and what ought or should be done. Bioethics is defined by Caplan (1997) as "the study of ethical issues in the life sciences and the distribution of scarce medical resources." Ethical decision-making involves careful consideration of difficult options (Aroskar, 1986; Arrant & Dimmitt, 1996). Indeed, ethical decision-making has been defined as the process of choosing between two (or more) equally unfavorable choices (Savage & Bever, 1989) or between two competing goods (Ballou & Bryant, 1997).

Deontological ethical approaches focus on the "rightness" or "wrongness" of an act that are determined by the obligations intrinsic to a role. These role-based duties and obligations provide the foundation for ethical codes espoused by health professions, including nursing. Normative ethics are dictated by the professional role. Although nurses approach ethical dilemmas from within a nursing context, difficulties may arise when the dilemma also involves other health care personnel, who may, in fact, have different duties and obligations. It is when the health care context itself provides conflict that the "rightness" or "wrongness" of a particular act becomes difficult to determine, potentially causing conflict among health care professionals. It is important to remember that nursing ethics emerge from a health care context that involves other professions.

HISTORICAL PERSPECTIVE

Early in the development of the nursing profession, the moral behavior of a nurse was judged on norms of value, that is, what is right or wrong *to be.* The first nursing code of ethics was expressed in the Nightingale Pledge (Peterson, 1987) which compelled the nurse to be devoted and virtuous. More informally, nurses were expected to be quiet, sober, and morally pure (Fowler, 1992). Deviations from these normative expectations often resulted in the end of one's nursing career.

As professional autonomy increased and the profession matured, nurses' ethical behavior focused on norms of obligation within the role: what is right or wrong *to do.* The "rightness" or "wrongness" of an act was judged on whether or not a nurse acted in the best interest of the patient and family. Several formal documents evolved which addressed these norms of obligation; one of these is the American Nurses Association ([ANA], 1985) *Code for Nurses with Interpretive Statements.* First developed in 1950, the ANA *Code* provided specific ethical guidance for nurses. The latest version of the *Code* (1985) is summarized in Table 15.1.

TABLE 15.1   ANA Code for Nurses (1985)

---

1. The nurse provides services with respect for human dignity and the uniqueness of the client unrestricted by considerations of social or economic status, personal attributes, or the nature of health problems.
2. The nurse safeguards the client's right to privacy by judiciously protecting information of a confidential nature.
3. The nurse acts to safeguard the client and the public when health care and safety are affected by the incompetent, unethical, or illegal practice of any person.
4. The nurse assumes responsibility and accountability for individual nursing judgments and actions.
5. The nurse maintains competence in nursing.
6. The nurse exercises informed judgment and qualifications as criteria in seeking consultation, accepting responsibilities, and delegating nursing activities to others.
7. The nurse participates in activities that contribute to the ongoing development of the profession's body of knowledge.
8. The nurse participates in the profession's efforts to implement and improve standards of nursing.
9. The nurse participates in the profession's efforts to establish and maintain conditions of employment conducive to high quality nursing.
10. The nurse participates in the profession's efforts to protect the public from misinformation and misrepresentation and to maintain the integrity of nursing.
11. The nurse collaborates with members of the health professions and other citizens in promoting community and national efforts to meet the health needs of the public.

Source: From Nurses' Association (1985). *Code for nurses with interpretive statements.* Kansas City, MO: Author. Used with permission. Copyright © 1976, 1985, ANA.

TABLE 15.2   Principles underpinning the ANA Code for Nurses (Harris, 1997):

Principle	Definition
Autonomy	Self-determination
Beneficence	Doing good
Nonmaleficence	Avoiding harm
Veracity	Telling the truth
Confidentiality	Respecting privileged information
Fidelity	Keeping promises
Justice	Treating people fairly

Note. From "Codes of Ethics and Scientific Integrity: What Relevance to Outcomes Activities," by M. Harris, 1997, *Advanced Practice Nursing Quarterly, 3,* p. 38. copyright 1997 by Aspen Publishers. Reprinted with permission.

ETHICAL PRINCIPLES

Ethical principles underpin the ANA *Code* (Harris, 1997), the most important of which is a fundamental respect for persons (ANA, 1985). The four cornerstone ethical principles include autonomy, beneficence, nonmaleficence, and justice; they flow from a principle-based ethics approach (Catalano, 1997; Gadow, 1983; Nelson, 1995; Wiens, 1993). These and other principles upon which the ANA *Code for Nurses* rests are briefly defined in Table 15.2; definitions of key concepts included in the *Code* are discussed elsewhere (Catalano, 1997).

NURSE INVOLVEMENT IN ETHICAL DECISIONS

Some nurse ethicists assert that nurses cannot autonomously make ethical decisions, while others believe that nurses must enjoy a high degree of autonomy in order to participate in ethical decision making (Aroskar, 1986; Cassidy & Oddi, 1988; Evans, 1986). Many nurses have not had the educational preparation necessary to handle the complex ethical dilemmas they encounter (O'Neil, 1991). Camunas (1994) reported that even some nurse executives (10%) were unfamiliar with the ANA *Code for Nurses.*

Greipp (1992, p. 734) said, "Most professionals agree on the need for ethical practice based on a code of ethics. The question becomes one of how to move professionals from this theoretical stance to assisting them to apply a theoretical code in practice." An ethical decisionmaking framework allows the advanced practice nurse to assist in data-gathering, identifying the appropriate principles involved, and to facilitate ethical discussions by providing a "systematic approach to ethical problems which are supported by sound reasoning and careful reflection" (Reeder, 1989, p. 2). Clarification of the pertinent, and often conflicting, principles and issues may also assist nurses in building sensitivity toward ethical decision-making (Aroskar, 1986; Fowler, 1989).

ETHICAL DECISION-MAKING MODELS

Ethical decision-making frameworks are diverse problem-solving models that contain multiple steps that allow a problem to be approached from a variety of disciplinary perspectives (Iris, 1995; Raheja, 1987). Typically, frameworks involve a data-gathering step and conclude with an evaluative step; however, intermediate steps vary widely. Further, the degree of complexity of the model often reflects the degree of complexity of a theory or theories that underpins it.

Advanced practice nurses (APNs) are often introduced to ethical decision-making frameworks during graduate education and discover the diversity of available models (Beauchamp & Childress, 1989; Catalano, 1997; Crisham, 1981; deMoissac & Warrock, 1996; Greipp, 1992; Hall, Glaser, & Harden, 1995). Integrating a model into advanced practice may be facilitated by the use of an accompanying framework. One such framework evolved after contemplation of a model developed by Thompson and Thompson (1985). Thompson and Thompson's model provides both depth and breadth of questions posed, allowing both principles of ethics and the context of decision-making to be identified and included. Although the framework reflects a nursing focus, it is flexible enough to be used by other heath care professionals. Since only a basic understanding of ethics is needed, the tool has been successfully used by students and staff nurses, as well as chaplains and medical residents. By using a pluralistic framework that is applicable to multiple disciplines, dialogue and collaborative decision-making may be enhanced (Nancy Green, personal communication, October 12, 1995). The decision-making model developed by the author, which is based on the model developed by Thompson and Thompson, is depicted in Figure 15.1.

Thompson and Thompson (1985) noted that the ethical decision-making process forming the foundation of the framework flows from principle-based ethics as well as moral reasoning, decision theory, and critical inquiry. Moral reasoning is defined as "the critical examination of a situation involving moral or ethical issues by analyzing, weighing, justifying, choosing and evaluating competing reasons for a given action" (Thompson & Thompson, p. 90). Critical inquiry involves analysis though which "asking proper questions" leads one to weigh choices thoughtfully. Further, decision theory, which arises from the discipline of mathematics, uses decision trees and algorithms to seek the "quantifiable solution to complex problems" (p. 90–91). Thompson and Thompson assert, however, that "the nature of bioethical decisions requires a blend of the analytical mind and caring heart" (p. 92), introducing the notion that a caring context underpins the ethical decision-making process.

Embedded within the model are underlying assumptions, that when explicated, may further illuminate processes involved. First, there is an assumption that the nurse can and will recognize an ethical dilemma. Second, moral reasoning, critical inquiry and decision-making occur all at once, when using the framework. Third, there is sufficient time to apply the process to a patient's situation. Fourth, there are several ethically congruent answers that can be described. Finally, the nurse has a sufficient understanding of ethical principles and appropriate Codes of Ethics to allow for ethical dialogue and assist in ethical decision making.

All of these assumptions and theories unfold within a caring, health-illness context of which nursing is a part, and is identified as a societal-based relationship with specific role requirements as outlined by the ANA *Code for Nurses* (1985). Further, collaboration and communication with others and critical reflection support the dialogic processes. An illustration of the processes, theories, and the overarching contexts involved when using the model is shown in Figure 15.1.

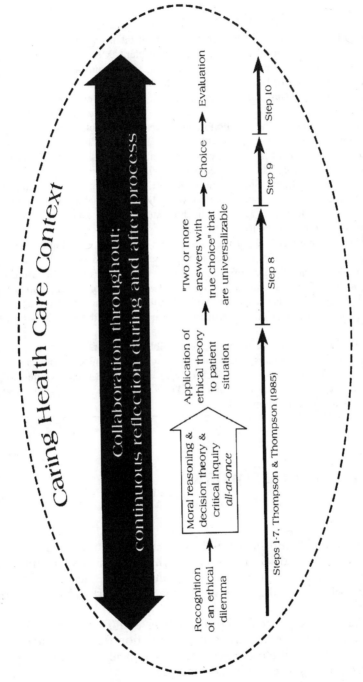

FIGURE 15.1 Decision-Making Model

Note: Adapted from J. Thompson and B. Thompson, 1985, *Bioethical decision-making for nurses.* East Norwalk, CT: Appleton-Century-Crofts.

TABLE 15.3　Case Study: Mrs. M.

Mrs. M., 41 years old, was admitted to a surgical intensive care unit (ICU) following her second failed kidney/pancreatic transplant. Mrs. M. is a resident of an East Coast city but is hospitalized in the Midwest, away from her family, because of the availability of a transplant center. Her husband must continue to work in order to maintain their health insurance. She has a 12-year-old son, Ben.

Mrs. M. has been critically ill for 6 weeks. She has diabetes and has experienced numerous complications. She is a double amputee. She is ventilator-dependent. She has had numerous infections. Medically, this gravely ill woman now needs a third kidney/pancreas transplant. She is in extreme pain; however she is receiving minimal pain medication for fear that these medications will interfere with Mrs. M. being weaned from the ventilator. She is semi-comatose, but does experience pain, as is evidenced by her facial grimaces when moved. She seems unable to make any decisions regarding her care. Mrs. M's health status is grave, and only a third kidney/pancreas transplant will save her life.

The primary nurse has brought the case of Mrs. M. to the attention of the APN following an extremely difficult night shift; the nurse wept in agony over caring for the patient and the anticipation of spending many more days or weeks caring for Mrs. M. in this difficult situation. The nurse states that caring for this patient constitutes an inappropriate use of resources and is wondering about the cost of the patient's care. But most of all, the nurse is concerned about the patients's quality of life.

There is minimal family or social support visible. However, when one walks into Mrs. M's room, cards, posters, and balloons from family members, friends, and Sunday school children cover every inch of wall space. Mr. M. calls frequently, but is rarely able to visit. Her husband and son know that she is seriously ill. Advance directives have not been completed.

USE OF THE FRAMEWORK

Thompson and Thompson's (1985) ethical decision-making framework can best be described within a context which uses a case to illustrate its application in practice. The case is introduced first and is followed by a discussion of each of the steps within the framework. The case is found in Table 15.3.

The framework proposed by Thompson and Thompson (1985) was used by this APN to reconstruct the information from the nurse and the patient's chart to initiate the dialogue for ethical decision-making that was requested in the consult she received.

STEP ONE: REVIEW OF THE SITUATION

In the first step, the situation is reviewed and includes the pertinent major events and concerns. This should be a brief summary of two to three paragraphs, rather than a detailed elaboration of the entire clinical course. Significant components of the situation are identified. Such questions as: "What are the health problems?" "What decisions need to be made?" and "What are the ethical and scientific components of the decision?" assist the APN in identifying pertinent aspects.

Next, the names of the individuals involved in the life and the care of the patient are noted: family members (their relationships and their loyalties), health care providers, and distant relatives. They are asked, "Who else is involved?" The APN can also include other persons, such as nutritionists or clergy. The APN must also consider whether similar patients might be involved in an indirect way. Information about the relationship of these individuals to the patient is obtained.

The question of who else may be involved is explored. Indirectly, the charge nurse, nursing management, and budget personnel may be affected. Also, other patients awaiting a kidney/pancreas transplant are included, as they will be directly affected by the decision to transplant this patient again. This patient was on the ICU at a time of high census. What about other others, such as patients awaiting surgery who will need critical care nursing skills and an SICU bed following their surgical procedure?

Step Two: Gather Additional Information

In this step, the nurse is prompted to gather additional information. Important background data such as demographics, social, economic, cultural, legal, and psychological information that might impact the ethical discussion are included. The health status of the patient and the significant others involved may greatly impact ethical decision making. These data are included to continue to build the documentation of the individual situation that comprise the contextual background for ethical decision making.

An assessment about the patient and family's ability to understand the situation is also a part of this step. Are there communication or cultural barriers which need to be bridged?

Step Three: Identify Ethical Issues

In Step 3, the nurse identifies the ethical issues at hand. This is a focus on ethical concerns, not clinical problem-solving. Appropriate language includes ethical and/or moral principles. It is at this step that the APN enters the science of ethics, using knowledge from philosophy and/or theology to assist in problem-solving. Usually, there is a reference to the historical roots of the problem. If necessary, ethical consultants can enter at this step.

Questions to ask include the following:

1. Will the third kidney/pancreas transplant be of benefit to Mrs. M.?
2. Can pain medications continue to be withheld in the small likelihood that her ventilator weaning may be accomplished soon?
3. Is a third kidney-pancreas transplant for this patient an appropriate use of the scarce and precious resources of organs?
4. Is continued critical care nursing an appropriate use of the scarce resources of the ICU?
5. Is the right to continued life the greatest good even if that prolonged life is one of intense, all-encompassing pain and suffering?
6. Of what concern is the quality of life for this patient and her family?
7. Is justice being supported through impartial decision making?
8. Does the end, prolongation of life, justify the means, excruciatingly painful curative efforts?

Step Four: Identify Personal and Professional Values

In this step, the focus of the discussion turns toward identifying those personal and professional values which may affect ethical decision-making. The clinical situation of the patient is not the focus of this discussion, but rather it is the ethical discussion which moves to the forefront. Ethical, rather than clinical, language is used. The health care provider asks, "What does my professional code of ethics say about this situation in light of ethical principles?" The nurse and/or other professionals reference the appropriate codes of ethics used in decision making. If multiple disciplines are involved, attention needs to be given to whether the ethical codes are congruent with one another.

Because many nurses use rules which emerge from their family of origin or their religious upbringing as aids in ethical decision-making (Camunas, 1994; Wagner & Ronen, 1996) it is important to capture these personal values within the framework. If religion, faith, or culture influence the decision, these principles are integrated in this section. Being clear about these personal influences assists others in understanding a particular ethical view and may also enhance dialogue among those involved in the process.

The ANA *Code* (1985) states that the most fundamental ethical principle is "respect for persons." This is actualized through preservation of autonomy, beneficence, nonmaleficence and justice. The code offers no specific rules or obligations on quality-of-life issues.

Personal and professional values of those caring for the patient are identified. The nurse caring for this patient was very clear that she felt a third transplant would only prolong the pain, suffering and, in the end, death of this patient. She also was fully aware that, without the transplant, the patient would surely die. "Respect for persons" in this case meant (for the nurse), preparing the patient and family for a comfortable death as being congruent with the obligation "to do no harm," or nonmaleficence. She also felt that the act of performing another kidney/pancreas transplant for this patient was an inappropriate use of scarce resources, also failing to support the utilitarian notion of the "greatest good for the greatest number of persons."

The physician teams were highly invested in this patient. Many scarce resources had already been used on the patient's behalf. The Hippocratic Oath compels physicians to provide benefit to patients whenever possible (Peterson, 1987). Physicians felt that another transplant should be offered to the patient once she became clinically stable enough to survive the surgery. Their rationale was that she was the most ill person on the transplant list.

Step Five: Identify Values of Key Individuals

The APN has the opportunity to identify the values of key individuals. Family members and key individuals are asked directly what values and beliefs they hold. Asking each family member directly, rather than assessing and assuming, prevents imposition of values on others and keeps all key players engaged in the decision-making process. Obtaining similar information from health care professionals is also done. It is important to clearly ask others the moral position and beliefs they hold. By focusing on the ethical principles identified in Step 3 and not on the clinical condition of the patient, all health care professionals' views can be considered and dialogue enhanced.

In the case of Mrs. M., the family was very active in their fundamentalist Christian church; indeed, the patient had been an active Sunday school teacher for years. The family espoused a strong leaning toward the preservation of life "at all costs." The patient did not have an advanced directive or other compelling statement of her treatment wishes which would have assisted the team in discovering and understanding her values and beliefs around these issues. Others involved in the care of Mrs. M. were deeply divided about the patient's condition and the numerous ethical implications. Ancillary team members' values reflected this range of values. Some supported the notion that a comfortable death was inherently a higher-quality existence than the torturous wait for complications to clear. Others agreed that life was worth preserving, regardless of the potential outcome. Ethical discussions near the bedside of this patient were frequently initiated; yet, the dilemma went unsolved as "doing nothing to decide" became the unintended and unconscious decision by default.

Step Six: Identify Conflicts in Values

Naming the conflict among values is a difficult but important step. Conflict is uncomfortable in some cultural groups, and also within the health care professional hierarchy, in which some professionals may hold more power than others (Arrant & Dimmitt, 1996). Nevertheless, it is important that conflicts are identified so that they may be discussed openly. Discovering when or why disagreements exist, and discussing these freely, may facilitate communication and ethical decision making.

Individual health care professionals are asked to identify conflicts within themselves. Conflicting loyalties and internal values are assessed. If possible, values are ranked, so that a clear picture of values and conflicts emerges.

Conflicts between key individuals are explored. Conflicts existed among those caring for Mrs. M. The family wanted all treatment to continue; however, they were not viewed as being aware of the day-to-day suffering experienced by Mrs. M. An uneasy resentment toward the family began to evolve because of the family's absence. It was known that Mr. M. needed to continue working in order to preserve critical insurance benefits for the patient.

Conflicts within the primary nurse were noted: she felt torn between her desire to advance the family's preferences and her own key values. She strongly valued the patient's, and by implication, the family's autonomy and rights to make informed treatment decisions. However, she also strongly valued the beauty of a comfortable death in which the patient is appropriately medicated for pain. She experienced a conflict between her need as a nurse to relieve suffering, a benefit to the patient, and the family's need to protect life at all costs. Mr. M. remained in conflict about his need to continue working and his deep and enduring desire to be at his wife's bedside during her critical illness.

Step Seven: Determine Who Should Decide

In this step the person who should be the ethical decision-maker is identified. By asking: "Who owns this problem?" and "Who decided who decides?" the APN begins to understand the complexity of ethical decision making. Determining "Who should decide" implicitly assumes that another is determining who has the final authority in ethical decision making. This is an ethically tenuous decision, as there may be inherent paternalism in determining who decides. Within nursing, the principle of respect for persons is supported when the individual patient decides. However, should the patient become incapable of making such a decision, then the process of determining who should decide is in itself an ethical decision.

For Mrs. M., this was an extremely difficult question. Because of the inability of the patient to make this decision herself, and because there was no written statement regarding her preferences, the family was supported as the decision maker. A telephone conference with Mr. M. and his son was arranged.

Step Eight: Identify the Range of Actions with Their Anticipated Outcomes

The team identifies all the possible outcomes, along with the ethical principles involved in each outcome. This step requires contributions

TABLE 15.4   Potential Treatment options for Mrs. M.

1. Place on the transplant list to be re-transplanted.
2. Continue the present treatment plan.
3. Modify the treatment plan by discontinuing dialysis but continuing the ventilatory support.
4. Modify the treatment plan by tapering life-support intravenous medications and discontinuing the ventilator.
5. Privately assist Mrs. M with suicide, even though it is against the law.
6. Do nothing.

from all key individuals. The APN, in collaboration with the primary nurse, may be able to identify several potential outcomes. Further consultation with the ethics team and the family and significant others involved (such as other health care professionals) may generate additional options. Collaborators ask, "What would happen if *this* were done?" Ethical theory, appropriate codes of ethics for professionals, and the Patient Bill of Rights all provide important input into the development of options.

This is a complex and lengthy process requiring identification of the full range of actions and their anticipated outcomes. All courses of action should be examined, using the ethical principles involved. The ethical action of doing nothing as nonintervention may have devastating personal and ethical consequences (Thompson & Thompson, 1985).

An important consideration in this step is the ethical principle of universality; in this principle, it is noted that any ethical decision which is made in fact impacts all others in the same or similar circumstance (Thompson & Thompson, 1985). Therefore, it is important to include the question: "What would happen to another patient in this situation if this ethical decision were implemented for her/him?" This allows society's interest to be brought into the issue and keeps intact the ethical issue of justice.

Numerous options were considered in the case of Mrs. M. These are shown in Table 15.4.

Step Nine: Decide on a Course of Action and Carry It Out (What is Done)

Considerable data were collected and much reflection occurred in relation to Mrs. M. Mrs. M.'s family came to see her. Both Mr. M. and Ben were aware of the amount of pain Mrs. M. was experiencing with every movement and every touch. A lengthy discussion of the ethical decision-making process was followed by a tearful declaration of choice by Mr. M to decline the option of a third transplant. This decision was made in consultation with other family members present at his side and by telephone. Dialysis was discontinued, and the use of pain medication greatly liberalized. As expected, Mrs. M. died within a few days with her loving family at her side.

Step Ten: Evaluation

It is important that those involved in ethical decision-making are provided with the opportunity to assess the results of the ethical action carried out in the previous step. The question posed is, "Was the outcome what was anticipated?" More importantly, "Did the action taken solve the ethical problem?" This prevents premature closure of the discussion and allows those health professionals involved to evaluate if another ethical decision needs to be made. Further, this step facilitates developing an understanding of the lessons learned in this specific situation. While it is understood that individual ethical decisions are not generalizable, the nurse identifies what information may be transferable to other situations.

CONCLUSION

It is important to see the embeddedness of ethical decision making in the clinical decision making and judicial decision-making processes. These processes can be intertwined and complex, making it difficult to achieve clarity in ethical decision-making. Also, it is noted that all of the options identified during the process reflect conflict among ethical principles and possible outcomes. Indeed, there is no single "right" answer, and all of the options presented in the eighth step were uncomfortable in at least some of the aspects. Yet, the dialogue resulting from the use of the Thompson and Thompson model (1985) allowed the APN, the primary nurse, the family, and others on the health care team to identify and describe the options, giving them ethical power through the development of voice.

Ethical frameworks assist the APN in decision making through identification of multiple, conflicting issues. Frameworks provide the opportunity for careful consideration of, and reflecting upon, complex patient situations and their impact. Nurses who use such frameworks for consultation in advanced practice settings may advance the role of nurses in the decision-making processes (Watson, 1993). Interdisciplinary discussions about individual cases facilitate education of health care professionals in the language and the philosophy of ethics.

Nursing ethics, at present, is embedded within the bioethical decision-making model that is the hallmark of medicine. Scholars continue to struggle with identifying nursing's unique ethical stance (Gadow, 1983; Noddings, 1984). There is ongoing debate among philosophers and nursing scientists regarding this issue, further challenging both clinical nurses and nurse ethicists.

Rather than simply reacting to ethical dilemmas, advanced practice nurses need to prepare for and initiate ethical discussions. This may be accomplished by carefully reflecting upon all aspects of the dilemma; clearly articulating values, beliefs and ideas; and accepting responsibility for decisions as they are made (Walleck, 1991). Nurses are called to think, reflect (Aroskar, 1986) and act (Holly & Lyons, 1993) in an ethically congruent manner.

REFERENCES

American Nurses Association. (1985). *Code for nurses with interpretive statements.* Kansas City, MO: Author.

Aroskar, M. (1986). Using ethical decision-making to guide clinical decision-making. *Pediatric Nursing Quarterly, 2*(2), 20–6.

Arrant, K., & Dimmitt, J. (1996). Choosing a framework for ethical analysis in advanced practice settings: The case for casuistry. *Archives of Psychiatric Nursing, 10*(1), 16–23.

Ballou, M., & Bryant, K. (1997). A feminist view of nursing ethics. *Critical Care Nursing Clinics of North America, 9*(1), 75–83.

Beauchamp, T., & Childress, J. (1989). *Principles of biomedical ethics.* New York: Oxford University Press.

Camunas, C. (1994). Codes of ethics as resources for nurse executives in ethical decision-making. *Journal of the New York State Nurses Association,* 25(4), 4–7.

Caplan, A. (1997). Bioethics: an introduction [On-line]. Available: http://www.med.upenn.edu/~bioethic/outreach/bioforbegin/beginners/html.

Cassidy, V., & Oddi, L. (1988). Professional autonomy and ethical decision making among graduate and undergraduate nursing majors. *Journal of Nursing Education,* 27(9), 405–10.

Catalano, J. T. (1991). Critical care nurses and ethical dilemmas. *Critical Care Nurse,* 11, 16–21.

Catalano, J. T. (1997). Ethical decision-making in the critical care patient. *Critical Care Nursing Clinics of North America,* 9(1), 45–52.

Clochesy, J., Daly, B., Idemoto, B., Steel, J., & Fitzpatrick, J. (1994). Preparing advanced practice nurses for acute care. *American Journal of Critical Care,* 3(4), 255–60.

Crisham, P. (1981). Measuring moral judgments in nursing dilemmas. *Nursing Research,* 30(2), 101–110.

Evans, M. (1986). Not free to be moral. *Australian Journal of Advanced Nursing,* 3(3), 35–47.

Fowler, M. (1992). Ethical decision-making in clinical practice. *The Nursing Clinics of North America,* 24(4), 955–65.

Gadow, S. (1983). Basis for nursing ethics: Paternalism, consumerism or advocacy? *Hospital Progress,* 64(10), 62–7.

Gadow, S. (1988). Covenant without cure: Letting go and holding on in chronic illness. In J. Watson, & M. Ray (Eds.), *The ethics of care and the ethics of cure: synthesis in chronicity* (Publication No. 15-2237) pp. 5–14. New York: National League for Nursing.

Greipp, M. (1992). Greipp's model of ethical decision making. *Journal of Advanced Nursing,* 17, 734–8.

Greipp, M. (1995). Culture and ethics: A tool for analyzing the effects of biases on the nurse-patient relationship. *Nursing Ethics,* 2(3), 211–20.

Harris, M. (1997). Codes of ethics and scientific integrity: What relevance to outcomes activities? *Advanced Practice Nursing Quarterly,* 3(3), 36–43.

Hill, M., Glaser, K., & Harden, J. (1995). A feminist model for ethical decision making. In Rave, E. J., & Larsen, C. C. (Eds.), *Ethical decision making in therapy: Feminist perspectives.* New York, NY: Guilford Press.

Holly, C., & Lyons, M. (1993). Increasing your decision-making role in ethical situations. *Dimensions in Critical Care Nursing,* 12(5), 264–70.

Iris, M. (1995). The ethics of decision-making for the critically ill elderly. *Cambridge Quarterly of Healthcare Ethics,* 4(2), 135–141.

Kachoyeanos, M., & Zollo, M. (1995). Ethics in pain management of infants and children. *MCN: American Journal of Maternal Child Nursing,* 20(3), 142–7.

de Massac, D. M., & Warnock, F. F. (1996). The evolution of caring within bioethics: Provision for relationship and context. *Nursing Ethics,* 3(3), 191–201.

Nelson, M. (1995). Client advocacy. In M. Snyder, & M. Mirr (Eds.), *Advanced practice nursing: A guide to professional development* (pp. 103–116). New York: Springer Publishing Company.

Noddings, N. (1984). Caring: A feminine approach to ethics and moral education. Berkeley: University of California.

O'Meary, A. (1989). Values, moral reasoning, and ethics. *Nursing Clinics of North America, 24*(2), 499–506.

O'Neil, J. (1991). Teaching basic ethical concepts and decision-making: A staff development application. *Journal of Continuing Education in Nursing, 22*(5), 184–8.

Peterson, S. (1987). Professional codes and ethical decision making. In G. Anderson, & V. Glesnes-Anderson (Eds.), *Health care ethics: A guide for decision makers* (pp. 321–9). Rockville, MD: Aspen.

Raheja, K. (1987). Jurisprudential inquiry model: A must for teaching nursing ethics. *Health Values, 11*(6), 35–40.

Reeder, J. (1989). Ethical dilemmas in perioperative nursing practice. *Nursing Clinics of North America, 24*(4), 999–1007.

Savage, T., & Bever, C. (1989). Ethical decision making models for nurses. *Chart, 86*(4), 2–5.

Self, D. (1987). A study of the foundation of ethical decision-making of nurses. *Theoretical Medicine, 8*(1), 85–95.

Smith, K. (1996). Ethical decision-making by staff nurses. *Nursing Ethics, 3*(1), 17–25.

Snyder, M., & Yen, M. (1995). Characteristics of the advanced practice nurse. In M. Snyder, & M. Mirr (Eds.), *Advanced practice nursing: a guide to professional development* (pp. 3–12). New York: Springer Publishing Company.

Thompson, J., & Thompson, B. (1985). *Bioethical decision-making for nurses.* East Norwalk, CT: Appleton-Century-Crofts.

Wagner, N., & Ronen, I. (1996). Ethical dilemmas experienced by hospital and community nurses: An Israeli survey. *Nursing Ethics, 3*(4), 294–304.

Walleck, C. (1991). Ethics: Building the framework for dealing with ethical issues. *AORN Journal, 53*(5), 1248–51.

Watson, C. (1993). The role of the nurse in ethical decision-making in intensive care units. *Intensive and Critical Care Nursing, 9*(3), 191–4.

Watson, R. (1987). Application of an ethical decision-making model. *Emphasis: Nursing, 2*(2), 92–100.

Wiens, A. (1993). Patient autonomy in care: A theoretical framework for nursing. *Journal of Professional Nursing, 9*(2), 95–103.

Chapter 16

ADVANCING YOUR CAREER IN THE HEALTH CARE MARKETPLACE

Jennifer Peters, Ph.D, RN

Changes in the health care system have and will continue to dramatically shape the careers of advanced practice nurses (APNs). The health-care marketplace of the 21st century presents distinct challenges and opportunities for APNs. Understanding and using principles of this marketplace will enable APNs to position themselves for successful and dynamic careers. This chapter addresses strategies that APNs can use to manage their careers and market themselves in an APN role.

HEALTH CARE SYSTEMS OF THE 21ST CENTURY

Prediction is at best an inexact science, particularly in the chaotic field of health care systems. But understanding the realities of the health care system will enable APNs to anticipate career opportunities and avoid significant career hazards. Over the next decade, the following characteristics of the United States health care system will likely affect the careers of APNs expanded efforts to reduce service costs (Brewer, 1997; Pew Health Professions Commission, 1995; Porter-O'Grady, 1997; Taylor, 1998):

- Consumer and payer demands for value and effective outcomes;
- Increased competition between providers for market share;
- Expansion of community-based health care services;
- Reduction in institutional care, particularly acute care services;
- Increasing focus on primary rather than specialized care;
  Expansion of capitated, subscriber-based systems;
- Growth of interdependent, rather than independent, practice models;
- Expansion of computer information systems for service delivery, outcomes analysis, and cost control; and
- Contraction of the job market, with increasing competition for available positions.

MAXIMIZING APN OPPORTUNITIES: A MARKETING APPROACH

Success in this competitive marketplace is dependent on the ability of APNs to deliver valuable services and to effectively market these services (Lachman, 1996). Marketing is determining what the customer wants or needs, designing a product/service to meet that need, and then communicating information about the product/service to potential customers (Gallagher, 1996; Lachman, 1996). The marketing process is guided by four concepts, the four Ps: Product, Price, Place, and Promotion. In addition, the potential customer, market segment, or target population of the marketing effort must be identified.

Depending on career stage, APNs target their marketing efforts to diverse prospective customers. During a job search, APNs market themselves and the APN role to potential employers. Current employers may be the focus of marketing to diversify services or achieve a job promotion. Consumers, the community, and other health care providers may be customers for entrepreneurial or independent practice ventures.

Characteristics of potential customers need to be examined. Geographic, demographic, economic, and psychosocial variables should be explored (Pakis, 1997). Sources of information on potential customers include census data, newspaper and media reports, employment offices of potential employers, needs surveys, focal groups, and personal contact with potential customers. The objective is to focus on the customers and let them identify the services they need and want (Lachman, 1996).

The first P of marketing—product—refers to the services APNs offer. Specific features of services including quality, outcomes, and options, need to be identified. Unique and special services should be highlighted to distinguish the product from that of competitors (Gallagher, 1996). Pricing, the second P of marketing, is often difficult. Once again, analyzing the competition and the current market through personal, informal contact is helpful. The third P—Place—refers to the geographic places and environment where the services are delivered. Convenience and access are important considerations related to place. Finally, the fourth P is promotion. Promotion, or selling a service, should only occur after the product, price, and place of the service have been identified.

SPECIFIC APN MARKETING STRATEGIES

Self-Inventory

Self-inventory and reflection are elemental components of APN career development, and must occur as precursors to the market plan. Critical, reflective questions to ask include:

- Who am I? What do I believe and value?
- Where and what do I come from?
- Where am I now?
- Where am I going and why in that direction?
- How will I get there?
- How will I know when I have attained my goals? (Neubauer, 1998, p. 3).

Price (1998) suggests the exploration of five points in self-reflection: abilities, interests, values, needs, and characteristics. Abilities can be analyzed through identification of skills, achievements, and failures. In addition to clinical/caregiving skills, APNs should consider abilities such as communication, teaching, consultation, research, leadership, organization, computer proficiency, mentoring, writing, political action and many others. Interests may be identified by listing those professional activities to which one is attracted or would like to do. Values are those principles or qualities that guide life and work. Listing and prioritizing values can clarify the relative importance of competing interests such as career, family, friends, and other demands.

Needs are identified by listing satisfiers and dissatisfiers in prior work situations. Levels of control, power, salary, independence, security, recognition, creativity, and achievement often appear on a list of needs. Finally, individual physical, emotional, and intellectual characteristics relevant to career and job performance should be listed. Factors such as physical limitations, endurance, stress tolerance, enthusiasm, creativity, sensitivity, knowledge level, and learning ability are but a few individual characteristics to inventory (Price, 1998). For APNs unfamiliar with self-inventory, detailed and helpful formats are available in the popular press (Bolles, 1997; Dawson & Dawson, 1996).

Knowledge Building

In addition to clinical knowledge, APNs must possess knowledge about professional issues, the health care needs of the community, and the marketing process. To successfully market oneself and the APN role, APNs must develop a working knowledge of:

- Regulations affecting advanced practice, including licensure, certification, prescriptive privileges, and collaborative practice;
- Reimbursement patterns and regulations;
- Health care services and unmet needs in the target market;
- The role and services of competitors in the target market;
- Communication skills, including professional networking and negotiation; and
- The target market's perception and utilization of APNs.

Developing an Ideal Job Description

For APNs seeking employment or promotion, developing a sample job description can be a helpful step in identifying and prioritizing the desirable attributes of a position. This job description provides a basis for informed negotiation during job interviews. Self-inventory, literature, and information from fellow APNs provide a basis to formulate the job description. It is important to be specific about desired job functions and job benefits. Specific dollar amounts should be attached to salary and monetary benefits. Specific amounts of time should be identified for vacation and leave time. Specific percentages of time spent in various job functions should be considered. Table 16.1 lists information to include in a sample job description (Bolles, 1997; Burke & Bair, 1998; Dawson & Dawson, 1996).

Developing a Career Portfolio

Career portfolios are personal files containing evidence of professional and academic achievement (Kelly, 1996). Development of the portfolio continues throughout an individual's career. The career portfolio is the resource from which documentation can be selected to use in marketing. Some individuals develop two types of portfolios—closed and open. The closed portfolio is personal, only viewed by the individual, and serves as the master file documenting career achievement. The open portfolio is used as a marketing tool and shared with potential employers and target markets. The open portfolio contains selected elements of the closed portfolio that are relevant to the current market. Open portfolios can be very powerful tools in the marketing or job search process because they demonstrate achievement and an organized approach to marketing (Bolles, 1997). Table 16.2 lists items that APNs may want to include in a closed personal career portfolio.

Because the APN role is new and often poorly understood in some potential markets, it is also helpful to maintain a master portfolio of documents describing and validating the APN role. Sharing this information with potential employers or markets can be very helpful. This portfolio includes research articles demonstrating the effectiveness of APNs; copies of APN practice regulations; and brochures from practice

TABLE 16.1 Elements of a Sample Job Description

Position functions and responsibilities
- Percentage of time (productivity expectations) for clinical care, client education, consultation, and research
- Usual and additional work locations
- Usual hours of work and on-call, weekend and holiday responsibilities
- Collaborative and independent responsibilities

Position qualifications
- Academic and continuing education
- Certification and licensure
- Professional experience
- Other (insurance, practice agreements)

Position in organizational structure

Performance evaluation
- Frequency
- Criteria for evaluation
- Evaluators

Salary range desired

Benefits desired
- Vacation days
- Sick days
- Paid holidays
- Retirement benefits (employer contribution, time required for vesting)
- Medical and dental insurance (individual and family coverage, fee-for-service or managed care, panel of providers, vision coverage, portability, pre-existing conditions coverage, pregnancy coverage, prescription coverage, long-term care options)
- Life insurance
- Short- and long-term disability insurance
- Malpractice insurance
- Licensing and certification fees
- Continuing education (travel, conference fees, meals, lodging)
- Orientation period (duration and content)
- Tuition reimbursement or waivers
- Professional dues
- Subscriptions to journals and texts
- Office, parking, computer, e-mail access, office supplies, medical supplies/ equipment
- Medical and clerical support personnel
- Answering service, pagers, and cell-phone
- Mileage reimbursement
- Interview and relocation expense coverage.

TABLE 16.2 APN Professional Portfolio

- Current resume and curriculum vitae
- Official transcripts of all academic programs post-high school
- Copies of nursing licenses and certifications
- Current list of references with addresses and phone numbers
- Malpractice insurance policies
- Records of continuing education attendance
- Reprints of publications
- Abstracts or brochures documenting conference presentations
- Newspaper or media recognition
- Evidence of honors or awards
- Prior references, recommendations, and evaluations
- A sample job description listing desirable job functions and benefits
- Examples of clinical achievements such as patient education programs/tools; history and physical examinations; quality improvement projects; and research utilization projects
- Professional organization memberships

organizations that document the role of APNs (American Nurses Association, 1993).

Resumés and Curricula Vitae

Resumés and curricula vitae (CVs) are powerful tools for individual marketing. An up-to date resumé and CV are essential components of the APN portfolio. They are used to communicate professional credentials to prospective employers, current employers, and colleagues. Both describe professional and educational accomplishments, but they differ in format and application.

Resumés are one- or two-page overviews of an individual's professional career. They are generally used to quickly advertise one's qualifications to potential employers, and brevity is important. There is no single, correct format for a resumé; it should be tailored to the prospective position. Functional resumés highlight areas of skill and expertise. Chronological resumés present the job history in chronological order. Critical information for any resumé includes name, address, phone num-

TABLE 16.3 Sample APN Resume

Maria R. Lewis, MSN, RN
2231 Echo Lane
St. Paul, MN 55105
(615) 222–2222

Objective	Gerontological Nurse Practitioner in a Community Setting	
Education	1998	University of Minnesota
		Minneapolis, MN
		Master of Science in Nursing
	1990	University of Michigan
		Ann Arbor, MI
		Bachelor of Science in Nursing
Experience	1995–present	Eastbrook Long-term Care Center
		Roseville, MN
		Clinical Coordinator
	1993–1995	Midwest Regional Medical Center
		Ann Arbor, MI
		Nurse Manager—Coronary Care Unit
	1990–1993	Midwest Regional Medical Center
		Ann Arbor, MI
		Staff Nurse—Coronary Care Unit
Licensure	RN, Minnesota	
Certification	Gerontological Nurse Practitioner, American Nurses Credentialing Center	
Honors/Awards	Gerontology Scholarship Award, University of Minnesota, 1997 Sigma Theta Tau, 1990	
Publications	Lewis, M. (1996). Assessing cardiac function in older adults. Long-term Care Nursing, 12, 221–223.	
Organizations	American Nurses Association Minnesota Gerontology Association	
Languages	Fluent in Spanish and French	
References	Available on request	

bers, e-mail numbers, fax numbers, education/degrees earned, professional employment, and licensure/certification (no license numbers). If space allows, selected information about publications, honors/awards, research/grants, presentations, teaching experience, consulting experience, membership in professional organizations, specific clinical or professional objectives, languages spoken, community service, or military service may be included. Information is often presented in reverse chronological order, with the most recent events being listed first in each category of the resumé. Table 16.3 shows a typical chronological resumé for an APN.

Curricula vitae are more lengthy descriptions of professional career and qualifications. They are often called academic resumés because of their use in academic settings. There is no maximum length for a CV; they will typically address all of the essential and additional information categories listed in the preceding discussion of resumés.

Most commonly, resumés and CVs are designed by APNs on a personal computer. Use of the personal computer enables updating as necessary. Books, journal articles, and software are readily available to guide those less familiar with the process. Helpful resources include Bolles (1997); Coxford (1998); Dawson and Dawson (1996); Markey and Campbell (1996); Straka (1996); and VGM Career Horizons (1998). Resumé design services are also available through professional printers.

The physical appearance of these documents is extremely important. They are often the first impression a potential employer has of an APN. A poorly designed resumé or CV may close the door to interviews with prospective employers. They should be neat, concise, well-organized, and visually appealing, with no errors in spelling or punctuation. High-quality paper should be used in printing. White or off-white paper with black print is most commonly used to give a traditional, professional appearance to the resumé or CV. It is helpful to have colleagues review and proofread these documents.

Information on resumés and CVs must be accurate and truthful. Many prospective employers define the information or format that should be used. Some things should not appear on the resumé or CV, including professional license numbers; names of references; salary expectations; and personal information, such as age, gender, ethnic background, height, weight, marital status, health status/disabilities, or Social Security Number.

When a resumé or CV is sent to a prospective employer, a cover letter should always accompany it. The cover letter introduces the APN as an individual to the prospective employer. It should be individualized to a position and express enthusiasm for future employment. The cover letter is direct, brief (no more than one page), and written in standard business format. Whenever possible, address the cover letter to a specific person. The letter should include the reason for writing and briefly highlight accomplishments. The previously suggested resources for resumé writing also have many helpful examples of cover letters. Table 16.4 is a sample cover letter to accompany an APN resumé or CV. It is important to follow up by telephone or mail on all resumés/CVs that have been sent to prospective employers. Follow-up indicates enthusiasm and persistence; two attractive qualities in potential employees. This communication should be initiated within two weeks of sending these documents.

TABLE 16.4   Sample APN Cover Letter

Maria R. Lewis, MSN, RN
2231 Echo Lane
St. Paul, MN 55105

September 1, 1998

Jane S. Parsons, Ph.D, RN
Director, Clinical Services
Gerontology Nurse Associates
3640 Simpson Street
Minneapolis, MN 55455

Dear Dr. Parsons:

We spoke briefly at the Minnesota Long-term Care Conference about a position for a Nurse Practitioner at Gerontology Nurse Associates. I am writing to express my interest in that position. I have recently completed my graduate nursing studies and have received my certification as a Gerontological Nurse Practitioner. I would like to pursue a career as a GNP in community and long-term care settings. My prior experience in long-term care and cardiovascular nursing provides me with an excellent background for this field.

    I have enclosed a copy of my resume for your review. I am interested in interviewing for the position and I can be reached at (615) 222–2222. Thank you for your consideration. I look forward to speaking with you.

Sincerely,
Maria R. Lewis, MSN, RN
Enclosure

Locating Opportunities

For most APNs, career opportunities do not just materialize; finding a great position is not just a matter of luck. Preparation, persistence, and personal contact are fundamental requirements.

    The US Department of Labor estimates that approximately 80% of all job positions are located through personal contacts or networks (Dawson & Dawson, 1996). Developing a network is not complex, but it does require the willingness to meet and communicate with new people. Every person the APN knows or knows of should be considered a potential contact. Helpful networks for APNs to explore include local professional organizations, other APNs already working in the same role, nurse managers in local health care organizations, faculty, and anyone else who may have knowledge of APN opportunities. Telephone contacts and personal meetings are both effective means of making contact. Informally meeting contacts over breakfast or lunch is a tried and true networking technique.

Traditional job search strategies should not be ignored. Weekly review of newspaper employment listings is important. In addition, professional journals often advertise for APNs. Mass mailings of resumés are generally not advisable, unless they are preceded by personal contact (Bolles, 1997). For APNs planning to use a professional job search firm, it is advisable to thoroughly research the track record of the firm and their experience/success in placing APNs.

Interviewing

Numerous books are written about job interviewing; but the essence of successful interviewing is not complex. Essentially, the interview is an opportunity for the applicant and the prospective employer to meet, to exchange information, and to evaluate whether or not a "fit" exists between them. Both parties are trying to determine if they have something to offer each other by exchanging very subjective information and cues.

In a competitive environment, APNs should expect to complete several interviews before locating an acceptable position. Typically, employers will utilize a series of interviews when hiring for APN positions. Applicants are screened in initial interviews. Follow-up interviews are scheduled for those applicants who successfully complete the screening. It is not unusual for an interview process to consume many weeks. Usually APNs will meet with several individuals from the organization during the interview process.

Interviewing requires homework. As previously discussed, APNs need to be informed about the characteristics of the organization. Physical preparation for the interview is also important—first impressions do count. Dress neatly and conservatively. Arrive for the interview on time. Bring copies of resumés and other supporting documents from the portfolio. Psychological preparation is essential. Nervousness during an interview is normal, but an ability to project self-confidence is important. For APNs unfamiliar with interviewing, Bolles (1997) offers detailed strategies for coping with interview anxiety. Anticipating questions that the interviewer is likely to ask and developing a list of questions to ask are two means of reducing the anxiety of interviewing (Coxford, 1998). Questions for APNs to ask during an interview are easily generated from the ideal job description. The following are questions typically asked of APNs in the interview process:

- What type of position are you interested in?
- Could you tell me about yourself?
- What are your strengths? Your weaknesses?
- What do you know about our company?
- What would you do in this situation (typical situation described)?
- Why are you leaving your present job?
- What are your professional/career goals?
- What do you enjoy most about work? Least? Why?
- Why should we hire you for this position?
- What salary do you expect?
- What questions do you have about this position? This company?

Federal law prohibits asking certain questions during the pre-employment interview. It is unlawful for an interviewer to ask about age, date of birth, children, age of children, race/ethnicity, religious affiliation, marital status, military discharge status, arrest records, home ownership, spousal employment, and organization/club memberships (Coxford, 1998; Dawson & Dawson, 1996). When these questions are asked, it is usually not out of malicious intent. However, it is best to prepare a gracious way of not providing an answer to such questions.

During the interview project a positive attitude, interest, and enthusiasm. Be friendly, smile, and make eye contact. Listen as often as speaking. Be professional in all interactions. Focus on the position, qualifications, and experience. Ask for the job. Thank the interviewer for the opportunity and ask when the hiring decision will be made. Finally, follow up with a written letter expressing thanks and continued interest in the position.

Negotiation and Employment Contracts

At some point in the interviewing process, the parties are likely to have different perspectives about the position, salary, or benefits. Negotiation is the process of resolving these differences. Negotiation should not be considered a win-lose, adversarial interaction. Rather, it is a win-win, or, some would suggest, a gain-gain situation for all parties (Laubach, 1997; Straka, 1997). Successful negotiation requires preparation, innovative thinking, integrity, respect for the other party, and superior listening skills (Straka, 1997). Negotiations should be focused on outcomes/results rather than emotions. The point of time to begin negotiation is after the prospective employer has expressed interest in hiring, but before the APN has agreed to take the job.

In the managed care marketplace, one of the most critical factors for APNs to understand and negotiate is the employment relationship (Cohen, Mason, Arsenie, Sargese, & Needham, 1998; Ecanow, 1995; Melby & Edmunds, 1997). It is imperative to be absolutely clear on whether the position is an independent contractor or an employee. In addition, critical questions about billing, primary provider listing, and productivity expectations need to be clarified. Finally, the level of independent control APNs have over practice issues such as ordering tests, diagnostic procedures, and specialty care requires attention.

As part of the negotiations, the issue of whether or not an employment contract will be used should be discussed. In the past, APNs were often hired based on an informal verbal contract and handshake. Today it is much more likely that APNs are asked to sign formal employment contracts or agreements. Employment agreements are legally binding contracts between employers and employees stating the terms of a working relationship. Employees hired without a contract are termed "at will" (Buppert, 1997). The employment contract provides for job security, as it limits the reasons for termination. "At will" employees may be terminated at any time without cause. In addition, the contract provides a vehicle to describe salary, benefits, productivity expectations, job functions, and hours of work. Before signing an employment contract, APNs should carefully review the contract, negotiate areas of confusion, and if necessary seek legal advice.

In particular, APNs should note covenants not to compete and termination clauses in the contract. A covenant not to compete is a contract clause that restricts an employee from practicing within a certain number of miles from an employer's business, for a certain period of time after the employee leaves the employer's business. Covenants not to compete are legal and enforceable if they are deemed reasonable by the courts. They protect the employer from APN competition in the event the APN leaves the employer. They restrict the ability of APNs to continue to practice in a geographic area. Table 16.5 contains an example of covenants not to compete. If possible, APNs should seek a contract that does not contain a covenant not to compete. If the employer insists on including the clause, APNs should seek a clause that is less restrictive in

TABLE 16.5   Contract Agreements and Clauses

Covenants Not to Compete

     Restrictive: "Upon termination of employment for any reason, the CRNA agrees not to practice within 50 miles of any present or future office of this practice for a period of 5 years."

     Less Restrictive: "Upon termination of employment for any reason, the CRNA agrees not to practice within 25 miles of the current office of this practice for a period of 1 year."

Termination Clauses

     Termination-with-Cause Clause:

     "The employer may terminate this agreement at any time by written notice to the CRNA for any of the following reasons:

         a) The CRNA dies or becomes permanently disabled;

         b) The CRNA loses his or her professional license;

         c) The CRNA is restricted by any governmental authority from rendering the required professional services;

         d) The CRNA loses his or her staff privileges;

         e) The CRNA conducts him or herself in a grossly negligent way."

     Termination-without-Cause Clause:

     "The employer may terminate this agreement at any time, for any reason, after giving the CRNA 30 days written notice."

---

terms of duration or geographic area (Blumenreich, 1996; Buppert, 1997; Ecanow, 1995).

     A typical employment contract will contain a termination section which will list events that are bases for termination of the employee "with cause." These events include loss of license/certification, gross negligence, death, or conviction of a felony. Some contracts include a termination "without cause" clause that states that the employee may be terminated at any time, for any reason with 30 days notice. Rarely should APNs sign a contract containing a termination "without cause" statement. It effectively removes the employee's job security that the contract provides. The only circumstance in which "without cause" termination would be acceptable is when the APN is unable to commit to the full duration of the contract (Buppert, 1997). Table 16.5 contains examples of "with" and "without-cause" termination clauses.

CAREER DEVELOPMENT THROUGH INNOVATION AND ENTREPRENEURIAL PRACTICE

Changes in the health care marketplace offer tremendous opportunity to innovative APNs. Visionaries see entrepreneurial and intrapreneurial opportunities for APNs in practice, management of APN services, public policy activism, research, and education. In addition, the changing characteristics of society in the 21st century lend themselves to new APN roles.

The essence of entrepreneurship is alertness to opportunities and the willingness to take innovative action to create benefit (Herron & Herron, 1991; White & Begun, 1998). The entrepreneur is typically self-employed or engaged in independent practice. The internal entrepreneur or intrapreneur innovates within the organization, typically as a salaried employee.

Entrepreneurs typically demonstrate expertise, the ability to deal with uncertainty, a willingness to take risks, high energy levels, a drive to succeed, and direction. They have a vision and are willing to act to achieve it (White & Begun, 1998). Success as an entrepreneur is dependent not only on personality, but on the availability of mentors who demonstrate the entrepreneurial process and can guide the new entrepreneur through successes and failures (Baker & Pulcini, 1990; Wilson, 1998).

It is risky to suggest entrepreneurial activities for APNs, because the truly innovative nurse will have begun to act far in advance of any publication. However, literature, societal trends, and characteristics of the marketplace give some indication of where entrepreneurial opportunities may exist for APNs. Clinical innovation is needed for the aging population; children and families affected by violence; persons dependent on drugs; preventive health care; persons living with AIDS; alternative and nontraditional therapies; vehicular trauma; ethnic groups; underserved groups in urban and rural areas; and symptom management—to name but a few. The literature suggests that APNs can establish innovative roles working as clinicians, researchers, educators, managers, leaders, activists, and product developers in a multitude of settings including industry; prisons; radio/TV/print media; government; insurance companies; acute-care; long-term care; home care; public health; managed care organizations; academia; and private practice.

REFERENCES

American Nurses Association. (1993). *Advanced practice nursing: A new age in health care.* Washington, DC: American Nurses Publishing.

Baker, M. M., & Pulcini, J. A. (1990). Innovation: Nurse practitioners as entrepreneurs. *Nurse Practitioner Forum, 1,* 169–174.

Blumenreich, G. A. (1996). Covenants not to compete. *Journal of the American Association of Nurse Anesthetists, 64,* 317–319.

Bolles, R. N. (1997). *The 1998 what color is your parachute.* Berkeley, CA: Ten Speed Press.

Brewer, C. S. (1997). Through the looking glass: The labor market for registered nurses in the 21st century. *Nursing and Health Care Perspectives, 18,* 260–269.

Buppert, C. (1997). Employment agreements: Clauses that can change an NP's life. *The Nurse Practitioner, 22,* 108–109, 112, 117–119.

Burke, C., & Bair, J. P. (1998). Marketing the role: Formulating, articulating, and negotiating advanced practice nursing positions. In C. Sheehy & M. McCarthy (Eds.), *Advanced practice nursing: Emphasizing common roles* (pp. 192–216). Philadelphia: F.A. Davis.

Cohen, S. S., Mason, D. J., Arsenie, L. S., Sargese, S. M., & Needham, D. (1998). Focus groups reveal perils and promises of managed care for nurse practitioners. *The Nurse Practitioner, 23,* 48, 54, 57–58, 60, 63, 67–70,76–77.

Coxford, L. M. (1998). *Resume Writing Made Easy.* Upper Saddle River, NJ: Prentice-Hall.

Dawson, K. M., & Dawson, S. N. (1996). *Job search the total system.* New York: Wiley.

Ecanow, M. A. (1995). Provider contracting: Avoiding the pitfalls by understanding the employment relationship. Journal of the American Association of Nurse Anesthetists, 63, 282–287.

Gallagher, S. M. (1996). Promoting the nurse practitioner by using a marketing approach. *Nurse Practitioner, 21,* 30, 36–37, 40.

Herron, D. G., & Herron, L. (1991). Entrepreneurial nursing as a conceptual basis for in-hospital nursing practice models. *Nursing Economics, 9,* 310–316.

Kelly, J. (1996). The really useful guide to portfolios and profiles. *Nursing Standard, 10,* 5–25.

Lachman, V. D. (1996). Positioning your business in the marketplace. *Advanced Practice Nursing Quarterly, 2,* 27–32.

Laubach, C. (1997). Negotiating a gain-gain agreement. *Health care Executive, 12,* 12–17.

Markey, B. T., & Campbell, R. L. (1996). A resume or curriculum vitae for success. *AORN Journal, 63,* 192–202.

Melby, C. S., & Edmunds, M. W. (1997). Negotiating the politics and policies of managed care. *AJN, Supplement 1997*, 2–7.

Neubauer, J. (1998). Personal development: A lifelong journey. *Advanced Practice Nursing Quarterly, 3*, 1–9.

Pakis, S. (1997). Managing the marketing function for advanced nurse practitioners in a managed care environment. *Seminars for Nurse Managers, 5*, 149–153.

Pew Health Professions Commssion. (1995). *Critical challenges: Revitalizing the health professions for the twenty-first century.* San Francisco, CA: UCSF Center for the Health Professions.

Porter-O'Grady, T. (1997). Over the horizon: The future and the advanced practice nurse. *Nursing Administration Quarterly, 21*, 1–11.

Price, J. L. (1998). A reflective approach to career trajectory in advanced practice nursing. *Advanced Practice Nursing Quarterly, 3*, 35–39.

Straka, D.A. (1996). Are you your resume? *Advanced Practice Nursing Quarterly, 2*, 75–77.

Straka, D. A. (1997). Negotiating in a new climate: Are you prepared? *Advanced Practice Nursing Quarterly, 3*, 88–89.

Taylor, D. (1998). Crystal ball gazing: Back to the future. *Advanced Practice Nursing Quarterly, 3*, 44–51.

VGM Career Horizons. (1998). *Resumes for health and medical careers.* Chicago: NTC/Contemporary Publishing Co.

White, K. R., & Begun, J. W. (1998). Nursing entrepreneurship in an era of chaos and complexity. *Nursing Administration Quarterly, 22*, 40–47.

Wilson, C. K. (1998). Mentoring the entrepreneur. *Nursing Administration Quarterly, 22*, 1–12.

INDEX

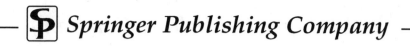

Springer Publishing Company

NURSES, NURSE PRACTITIONERS
Evolution to Advanced Practice
Third Edition
Mathy D. Mezey, EdD, FAAN, RN and
Diane O. McGivern, PhD, FAAN, RN, Editors

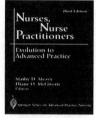

*This third edition provides pathways of understanding, appreciation, and
direction as the APN forges ahead into the twenty-first century."*
                          –From the Foreword by **Loretta C. Ford**, RN, EdD, FAAN

This textbook introduces advanced practice nursing students to the
practical information they will need to work in today's health care
arena. It examines all facets of the APN role with an emphasis on
nurse practitioners and primary care. New to this edition are chapters on
managed care, the acute care nurse practitioner, Medicare
reimbursement and payment issues, and more. The book contains
numerous personal essays describing first-hand experiences in
the field, by both nurses and their physician colleagues. Contributors
include Claire Fagin, Eileen Sullivan-Marx, and Patricia Barber.

> **Partial Contents:** Historical, Educational, Research and Philosophical
> Perspectives • Preparation and Clinical Practice • Research in Support
> of Nurse Practitioners • Philosophical and Historical Bases • The
> Practice Arena • Primary Care as an Academic Discipline • Family
> Nurse Practitioner in Urban Family Practice • Surgical Intensive Care
> Unit • Practice with Pateints with HIV/AIDS • Physician and Nurse
> Practitioner Relationships • Evolving Models of Advanced Nursing
> Practice • Nurse-Midwifery and Health Care for Women • Meeting the
> Needs of Older Adults for Primary Health Care • Academic Nursing
> Practice: Power Nursing for the 21st Century • Legislation, Law, and
> Reimbursement • State Nurse Practice Acts

Previous edition won 2 AJN Book of the Year Awards
Nurse's Book Society Selection

       1999   464pp.   0-8261-7771-9   hardcover   www.springerpub.com

536 Broadway, New York, NY 10012-3955 • (212) 431-4370 • Fax (212) 941-7842

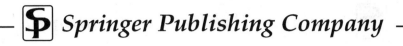 *Springer Publishing Company*

The Acute Care Nurse Practitioner

Barbara J. Daly, PhD, RN, FAAN, Editor

"★★★★!" I highly recommend this book for all individuals involved in the ACNP movement."
—**Doody Publishing, Inc.**

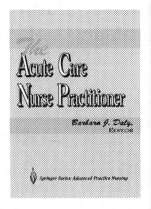

This book describes the rapidly emerging role of the nurse practitioner in the acute-care hospital setting. It also provides guidelines for educators involved in starting Acute Care Nurse Practitioner (ACNP) programs, for administrators considering hiring ACNPs, and for ACNPs themselves as they prepare for practice. The book outlines priorities in the initial development of a new specialty: defining the mission of the ACNP, designing and implementing educational programs, finding a role for the ACNP once they are educated, and describing practice models. This pioneering publication will be of interest to nurse practitioners, educators, and health care administrators.

Contents: Introduction: A Vision for the Acute Care Nurse Practioner Role • Development of the Acute Care Nurse Practitioner Role: Questions, Opinions, Consensus • Influence of the Health Care Environment • Educational Standards for ACNPs • Acquiring Clinical Skills and Integrating into the Practice Setting • An Administrative Perspective on the Acute Care Nurse Practitioner Role • Actualization of the ACNP Role: The Experience of University Hospitals of Cleveland

AJN Book of the Year Award
Brandon/Hill Selected List of Nursing Books 1997

1997   192pp.   0-8261-9480-X   hardcover   www.springerpub.com

536 Broadway, New York, NY 10012-3955 • (212) 431-4370 • Fax (212) 941-7842